Drugs and the Inheritance of Behavior

A Survey of Comparative Psychopharmacogenetics

Drugs and the Inheritance of Behavior

A Survey of Comparative Psychopharmacogenetics

P. L. Broadhurst

University of Birmingham
Birmingham, England

PLENUM PRESS · NEW YORK AND LONDON

Library of Congress Cataloging in Publication Data

Broadhurst, Peter Lovell, 1924-
   Drugs and the inheritance of behavior.

   Includes index.
   1. Psychopharmacology. 2. Pharmacogenetics. 3. Behavior genetics. I. Title. [DNLM:
1. Pharmacogenetics. 2. Behavior—Drug effect. 3. Psychotropic drugs—Pharmaco-
dynamics. QV38.3 B863d]
RM315.B67   615'.78   78-3617
ISBN 0-306-31105-4

© 1978 P. L. Broadhurst

Published by Plenum Press, New York
A Division of Plenum Publishing Corporation
227 West 17th Street, New York, N.Y. 10011

Printed in the United States of America

Preface

The title of any monograph must necessarily be a compromise between brevity and precision, and the needs of this compromise are particularly pressing in a newly emerging area of scientific interest, one that is not only inter- or bidisciplinary, but tridisciplinary, involving as it does psychology, pharmacology, and genetics. The temptation to call this work "psychopharmacogenetics"—*tout court*, if the phrase can be applied to so polysyllabic a construction—was removed by the timely appearance of the book under that title edited by Eleftheriou (1975*b*). Accordingly, something less novel has been chosen. It might be thought to promise more than it delivers and to delineate a wider field than it covers, but I have sought to add a corrective degree of precision in the subtitle which accurately defines what is intended even at the cost of further polysyllabification.

The survey of a disparate field of this kind entrains difficulties that go beyond what to call it. The claims of the parent disciplines for methodological supremacy are strong and difficult to resist. What I have done is to seek to impose a degree of coherence on the chosen area by always inquiring to what extent a particular methodology, derived from one part of one of them only, can be applied to the whole. This is biometrical genetics, which has had conspicuous success in its application to that area of plant genetics for which it was developed and has further demonstrated its power in its applicability to behavior, first at the animal level and more recently at the human level as well. The present extension to psychopharmacology represents a new challenge: The reader must judge the extent to which its success has made the enterprise worthwhile.

The preparation of this work was supported by a grant from the Medical Research Council of Great Britain in aid of research in psychogenetics to Professor J.L. Jinks, F.R.S., and the author. It was also greatly furthered by my Resident Fellowship during 1973 and 1974 at NIAS (Netherlands Institute for Advanced Study).

It is a pleasure to acknowledge the friendly stimulation of Giorgio Bignami, and the kindness of the following colleagues in commenting on various parts of this monograph: H. Anisman, D. W. Bailey, D. A. Booth, D. A. Buxton, R. Dantzer, B. E. Eleftheriou, K. Eriksson, H. J. Eysenck, D. W. Fulker, J. L. Fuller, J. L. Jinks, A. Oliverio, C. W. T. Pilcher, D. J. Sanger, K. P. Satinder, K. Schlesinger, R. A. Shephard, I. Stolerman, P. A. Tyler, and J. H. F. van Abeelen.

Finally, K. J. Drewek, E. F. Gouthwaite, Barbara Bates, and my children, Tom and Eleanor Broadhurst, have at various times assisted mightily with bibliographic matters, and Chris Benkwitz and Sandra Cumberland have efficiently seen me through several drafts. But, as always, the greater debt of gratitude I owe is to Anne, my wife and close colleague.

P. L. Broadhurst

Birmingham, England

Contents

Chapter 1

Introduction

This chapter is concerned with the definition of the subject matter of this book and the context in which it appears. Pharmacogenetics, as such, may be generally understood to cover the whole range of reactions to drugs as modified by genetic determinants, whether those reactions occur in animals or in humans and whether they are regarded as physiological or behavioral. Fuller (1970*a*, Fuller and Hansult, 1975) has rather briefly reviewed the field in the latter sense: On the other hand, Meier's monograph (1963), while restricted to animals, emphasizes physiology and biochemistry, especially stressing genetic pathology in that the effects of hereditary disorders of function on drug response are prominently considered. Others reviewing the area, for example Kalow (1962) and Vesell (1975), have also concentrated on unusual responses to drugs, especially in humans. Green and Meier's (1965) brief but genetically sophisticated review largely deals with physiological variables, and Sprott and Staats (1975) cover psychopharmacology in their useful bibliography. Eleftheriou (1975*c*) in his introduction to the valuable set of contributions which he edited, many of which will be cited separately in later chapters, sought to define psychopharmacogenetics thus: ". . . the area which is being specifically created in this presentation is an area which deals with pharmacologic agents that alter a given behavior in controlled genetic systems" (p. 1).

The emphasis in this work is somewhat different, and is perhaps closer to that of Dantzer (1974), who may have been the first to use the term psychopharmacogenetics—albeit in French—in the preferred sense. Just as psychogenetics is the genetics of psychological, that is, behavioral functions—behavior genetics is, in fact, what it is most frequently termed—and

1

psychopharmacology is often conceived of as the study of the effects of drugs on behavior, psychopharmacogenetics is the genetical analysis of behavior as modified by drugs—the genetics of drug responsivity as measured by behavioral methods. It is not, in my view, necessarily limited to controlled genetical systems, though genetical analysis naturally proceeds more expeditiously in such circumstances. The drug response may be observed in the behavior of any population or sample of a population of organisms: Techniques for the analysis of a response observed under such circumstances exist, though to my knowledge they have not as yet been applied.

Hence, here we are concerned only with essentially normal behavioral reactions to drugs in nonhumans—comparative psychopharmacogenetics, in a word (or two!)—and our consideration of the literature, like earlier ones (Broadhurst, 1964, 1977), will be centered in this area to the exclusion of more than passing reference to other topics.

A second matter in relation to the subject of the present chapter is the nature of the response to be observed in a psychopharmacological (as in any other psychological) experiment, and how it can be causally analyzed. Behavior is rarely the outcome of heredity as such, or of environment either: It is the multidetermined end product of often complex genetic and environmental determinants whose effects summate. Neither is directly observable and their influence can only be assessed via their effect on the phenotype, that is, that aspect of the organism which is being observed or measured. This view can be summarized in the fundamental genetical equation

$$\text{Phenotype} = \text{Genotype} + \text{Environment}$$

which is as applicable to behavior as to any other aspect of the phenotype, and to behavior as modified by drugs as much as to any other change induced by stimuli in the environment. That the stimulus here is a change in the internal milieu of the organism is irrelevant; it is nonetheless environmental, just as, for example, a dietary manipulation or brain lesion would be. This view stems partly from the genetical definition of environment by exclusion as being all those influences occurring after the moment of conception when gametic fusion determines individual genotype irrevocably for the life of the organism. Thus it is that prenatal effects are, by this rubric, environmental, even though they may be constitutional in that they are present at birth and endure throughout life. Moreover, drug effects are, in general, macroenvironmental in the sense that they are usually the consequence of deliberatley imposed environmental treatments, often in the context of an acute experiment, and hence to be contrasted with microenvironmental variation, which subsumes all adventitious and uncontrolled variation consequent upon the individual life history of the organism, especially husbandry in the case of laboratory animals. Vesell *et al.* (1976) illustrated the subtlety of such effects by showing that, for instance, aromatic hydrocarbons from bedding, ammonia from sanitary trays, and contaminants in the water supply can all be implicated in strain differences in chloroform toxicity in mice.

In this way we can see that the externally observable behavioral response to a drug can be viewed as a property of the phenotype like any other, and amenable to analysis by methods appropriate to the study of the inheritance of behavior. In general, behavior shows a metrical quality, like stature, rather than displaying discrete types, like blood groups, and the classical Mendelian analysis has been modified accordingly to cope with quantitative variation of this kind. Hence methods such as those of biometrical genetics (Mather and Jinks, 1971) which assume the operation of a large number of genes acting additively (or subtractively) in relation to each other and to the environment have proved especially suitable in psychogenetics. Some stress will therefore be laid on this approach in what follows, but not to the exclusion of the discussion and evaluation of other methods where they have been shown to be applicable.

Otherwise the application of genetical techniques to psychopharmacological phenotypes has followed relatively conventional lines: Attempts at selective breeding and the study of strain differences, followed by the analysis by means of inbred strains and crosses between them, including the search for the effects of major genes, almost always using standard laboratory animals, have all been prominent. This survey will be organized on the basis of the utilization of these techniques, but with one exception that relates to sex differences—a genetical variable *par excellence*, but one not always recognized as such—and it is with a consideration of the psychopharmacology of sex differences that we begin.

Chapter 2

Sex Differences

Sex differences in drug responsivity are generally not studied for their own sake. In this respect they resemble species differences, another important class of genetically determined responses, which are nevertheless outside the scope of this review [see Brodie (1962) and Ellinwood and Kilbey (1975) for surveys, and Karczmar and Scudder (1969) and Richardson *et al.* (1972) for contemporary examples described in Sections 7.3 and 5.2, respectively]. Indeed, effort is often made to exclude sex as a potentially disturbing variable by using subjects from one sex only—usually males. The rationale here is that tacitly applied in much behavioral experimentation, that is, the need to avoid possible artifacts arising from differences in general activity associated with the estrus cycle of females. The evidence for such contamination remains slender, though the basic proposition that females of laboratory rats show differential general activity associated with stage of estrus is reasonably secure (Finger, 1969). That some caution is appropriate can be justified by reference to work such as that of Whitman and Peretz (1969) who showed that the peak of activity in the female rat associated with ovulation can be delayed by an injection (30 mg/kg) of sodium pentobarbital.

However, there are many experimental situations in psychopharmacology in which such detailed considerations as are involved in the recognition of estrus phase are inappropriate or inoperative, and in which there is no special reason for suspecting sex differences in dependent variables. In such cases, the inclusion of animals from both sexes—females as well as males—can well be justifed by considerations relating to the efficiency of experimental design, including animal utilization, since, if no sex

5

difference is in fact detected then the size of the experiment is doubled, with a consequent increase in the probability of obtaining reliable results. The alternative outcome—the finding of differences attributable to sex where none were expected—is itself of sufficient scientific interest, even if serendipitous and unsought, to merit attention.

Thus most of the work on sex differences has been incidental rather than deliberate in that it has been the result of experimentation designed for other purposes, and so it is that studies concentrating on sex differences as the main or a major outcome are relatively rare in psychopharmacology, and those setting out explicitly to study them even rarer. Among the former, the following may serve as examples. Greenough and McGaugh (1965) found that the facilitatory effect of strychnine sulfate administered immediately after two learning trials in a Lashley III maze—as opposed to administration before the trials or after a five-day delay—was somewhat greater among females of the Sprague–Dawley strain of rats used than males. The authors note (p. 293) that "the results clearly point to a greater drug–sex interaction than has been found in similar experiments. . ." (e.g., McGaugh *et al.* (1962*b*), but since they do not evaluate this interaction statistically, only nonparametric tests having been applied to between-treatment comparisons with no between-sex comparisons being reported, this conclusion remains speculative. Another study reporting major differences according to sex was that of Bradley *et al.* (1968), in which the exploration of holes ("head dipping") by mice of an inbred strain was observed under the effects of amphetamine sulfate, or of amylobarbitone sodium,or of a mixture of the two, all in various doses. Analysis of variance of the difference between drugged mice and saline-injected controls gave a sex difference that was significant at the 1% level. The direction of the difference was not stated, but it can be seen from a graphical comparison that males were characterized by a greater susceptibility to the depressive effect of amylobarbitone and had a somewhat lower response, on the average, to the stimulant effects of both amphetamine and the mixture, which suggests that a drug–sex interaction was present. The reported absence of any such significant differences on a retest a week later, for which no drugs were given, suggests differential retention between the sexes. Satinder and Petryshyn (1974) note a greater depression of one-way avoidance conditioning performance of female rats of a selected strain under a large (4.0 mg/kg) dose of amphetamine (Experiment 1), and evidence suggestive of sex differences interacting with strain is presented by Russell and Stern (1973) in the preference of rats for alcohol as opposed to water, and by Hatchell and Collins (1977) in the activity response of mice to nicotine. An investigation that made specific provision for sex differences in its analysis was that of Robustelli (1966) on the effect of nicotine on avoidance conditioning in mice, though the differences found were not significant. Other reports of work which, it is judged, would have adequately permitted the establishment of sex differences—had they been present—in drug response include those of Anisman (1975*a*), Eriksson and Kiianmaa (1971), Fleming and Broadhurst (1975), Gupta and Gregory (1967), Gupta and Holland (1969*a*), Henry and Schlesinger (1967), Huff (1962), Poley and Mos (1974), Powell *et al.* (1967), Richardson *et al.* (1972), Satinder (1971, 1972*a,b,* 1975, Experiment 2, 1976, 1977*a*, Experiment 2, 1977*b*), Schlesinger *et al.* (1968*a*), Stasik and Kidwell (1969), and Westbrook and McGaugh (1964). Others report overall sex differences, though not involving an interaction of sex with response to a drug: They include Baer and Crumpacker (1975), Brewster (1969), Burt (1962), McGaugh and Thomson (1962), and Vesell (1968).

Of studies specifically designed to analyze the effect of sex as a determinant of response to drugs, the work of Wallgren (1959) is a good example. He studied the effects of ethanol on motor incoordination in rats by means of the tilting plane test which, as the name implies, involves measuring the angle at which the animal begins to slide down a plane when it is gradually tilted from the horizontal toward the vertical. He showed that the males had a lower threshold of response, which could not be attributed to any sex differences in blood alcohol or its rate of oxidation—there were none—but which may have been occasioned by hormonal effects or differences in the rate of learning, since the subjects were tested six times on the tilting plane.

From the same laboratory, Eriksson and Malmström (1967) reported sex differences in preference for alcohol* among a Wistar strain of rats. Careful experimentation over a prolonged period (six weeks) allowed the firm conclusion to be drawn that females voluntarily drink more than do males of an aqueous solution of 7.9% ethanol wt./vol. (equals 10% vol./vol.) when a free choice between the solution and tap water was offered to the two sexes. Analysis of the differences between them in other measures of fluid and food intake, body weight, and metabolism allowed the authors to resolve the discrepancies in the reports in the literature, which

---

*Whether or not alcohol preference in laboratory animals is based on a pharmacological action of the drug or merely represents either a nutritional or a perceptual response to it, such as taste, is a moot point and depends on the nature of the as yet unelucidated mechanisms that initiate and sustain it. For example, Nachman's (1959) work, based on a successful selection experiment for saccharin preference, has been excluded on the latter grounds, but it is difficult to know if similar considerations apply to preference for alcohol, and consequently whether it falls outside the scope of this book in the way it has also been decided that—though for different reasons—treatment by the use of exogenous hormones does. But without prejudice to the answers to the etiological problems, it has been decided to include the psychogenetics of alcohol preference in animals in the present review, especially because of the important contributions that have been made to the topic by work using this drug.

TABLE I
Psychopharmacology of Sex Differences

Reference	Subjects	Drug	Measure	Outcome
Greenough and McGaugh (1965)	Sprague-Dawley rats	Strychnine sulfate immediately after learning	Lashley III maze	Facilitated females
Bradley *et al.* (1968)	Inbred mice	Amphetamine sulfate and/or amylobarbitone sodium	Head dipping	Males more susceptible to amylobarbitone depression; less response to amphetamine and mixture
Satinder and Petryshyn (1974)	Selected strain rats	Amphetamine	One-way avoidance	Females more depressed
Hatchell and Collins (1976)	Mice	Nicotine	Activity measure	Sex differences varied with strain
Masur and Benedito (1974*b*)	Rats	Apomorphine	Dominance in food seeking	Female became dominant
Wallgren (1959)	Rats	Ethanol	Tilting plane motor coordination	Males lower fall threshold
Eriksson and Malmström (1967)	Wistar rats	Ethanol	Preference	Females greater
Eriksson and Pikkarainen (1968, 1970)	C57BL and CBA mice	Alcohol	Preference	Females greater
Russell and Stern (1973)	Rats	Alcohol	Preference	Sex difference varied with strain

they surveyed, about the existence or even the direction of sex differences in alcohol preference in rats, as well as in mice and hamsters, in the following way: ". . . the females voluntarily. . . drink more alcohol than the males. But in situations where the rats on free choice consume very small amounts of alcohol, it may prove impossible to demonstrate a sex difference. The total ability to consume will then never be mobilized and alcohol as a calory source will play an insignificant role, which is almost equal in the two sexes. . . . We assume that this sex difference in voluntary alcohol consumption can be found in all rat strains where the weight differences between the sexes is large enough and where the animals voluntarily drink large amounts of the alcohol solution" (Eriksson and Malmström, 1967, p. 391).

This conclusion is to some extent validated by studies on mice by Eriksson and Pikkarainen (1968, 1970) in which two inbred strains (black and albino, C57BL and CBA, respectively) were compared and it was found that among the former, which showed a relatively greater preference for a 7.9% (wt./vol.) ethanol solution over water, there was a markedly greater female alcohol intake. In the second report the same two strains were used and the earlier findings confirmed. In addition, it was shown that among a crossbred generation derived from the two strains, where the overall intake was considerably lower, there was only a very small and probably non-significant difference in favor of the females.

An interesting attempt to use a sex difference to elucidate drug action was reported by Masur and Benedito (1974*b*) who found that the usual tendency for females to lose to males in a food-seeking situation in which the runway to the goal was too narrow to allow them to pass in opposite directions could be significntly modified by 1.0 mg/kg of apomorphine. However, the authors concede that the possible relationship of the behavior observed to the effect of the drug in stimulating dopamine receptors in the brain is not established.

As may be seen from this doubtless selective review of the psychopharmacological work reporting sex differences in animals, summarized in Table I, there are a few if any generalizations which flow from it. The volume of work is as yet insufficient to attempt even the broadest generalization of the kind that, for example, females of a particular species are behaviorally more susceptible than males to drugs of a certain class. The only instance in which we can point to the possible foundations for such a statement is in work suggestive of a sex difference in alcohol preference.

This being the state of affairs, it is not surprising that no approximation to genetical analysis of the effect of sex chromosomal differences has been encountered. No instances of sex linkage or sex limitation of gene action on drug response as a phenotype can be cited, and it seems that until some of the more basic and straightforward requirements for relatively simple genetic analysis can be met it will be unlikely that the more complex analyses required for demonstrating sex differences can be undertaken.

Chapter 3

Pharmacogenetical Selection

In psychology, and in genetics itself for that matter, much effort has been put into selective breeding as a technique for the study of inheritance. Tryon's deservedly famous psychogenetic experiment of the 1920s and 1930s in which rats were selected bidirectionally for speed of acquisition of maze learning led to the foundation of the *Tryon maze-bright* and *maze-dull* strains, now known as TMB and TMD, respectively, descendants of which are still in use, as we shall see. However, while the process of selection itself is valuable both for the demonstration of the importance of genetic influences that a successful selection experiment provides and for the utility in other respects of the resultant strains—usually two—which emanate from it, it is not especially well suited to the fine-grain analysis of genetical and environmental determinants of the phenotype of interest and of their possible interaction. More efficient techniques are available in the study of established strains and the crosses between them, though such strains may, of course, themselves be the product of behavioral, or other, selection experiments. Moreover, "efficiency" here specifically includes the amount of effort involved in addition to the accuracy of the analysis, for selective breeding is an arduous and lengthy technique involving a considerable investment of resources over a relatively prolonged period.

It is not surprising, therefore, that the technique has not been widely applied in psychopharmacology and indeed only a few studies have been reported in which selection for a phenotype relating to drug response has been at all successful. The first to be considered here is the Finnish Alko Research Laboratories' study of selection in the rat for high and low ethanol preference. In view of the importance of this study a detailed

11

description of the techniques employed is in order, since it will serve as an orientation to other selections for drug responses in rats and mice and to the several further selection studies for other behavioral variables in rodents, some of which have been quite widely used in psychopharmacology.

Eriksson's (1969*b*) monograph supplements other reports (e.g., Eriksson, 1965, 1974, 1975; Eriksson and Narhi, 1973) on the establishment of the two strains, which have since been renamed the AA (*A*lko *A*lcohol) and ANA (*A*lko *N*on*a*lcohol) strains of rats (Eriksson, K., 1972*b*; Eriksson, C. J. P., 1973), a nomenclature avoiding the earlier use of the term "addiction," which was agreed to be potentially misleading. The system of lettering used is based on that used for designating inbred mouse and other rat strains (Festing and Staats, 1973), which is coming to be adopted also for selected rat strains, whether inbred or not. It refers by initial letters to the original location of the strains, or in special cases, as in the Tryon strains mentioned above, honors their founder and indicates the phenotypic differences involved.

The monograph reports on the development of the strains to the eighth generation of selection (S_8). The phenotypic measurement on which further breeding for each subsequent generation was based was taken when the rats were three months old. First came a 10-day habituation period in which two standard drinking bottles, both containing a 7.9% (wt./vol.) solution of absolute alcohol in tap water, were provided in the individual cage in which the rat was housed in order to habituate the rat to the taste of alcohol; that is, ethanol intake was forced. Following this stage of the experiment, a four-week free-choice period was given, during which one only of the two bottles held the solution, the other providing tap water only, and the position of the two was interchanged at least once a week. Some 25% of each generation were selected for further breeding on the basis of their high or low preference scores, that is, the proportion of the total liquid consumption represented by the volume of alcohol consumed, expressed as a percentage. This is a measure that is susceptible to disturbance if the total level of liquid intake varies, and so for other purposes another measure, intake of alcohol calculated as consumption per unit of body weight, is preferred. But under the carefully controlled environmental conditions operating here—essential in any selection experiment that seeks to maximize a genetic as opposed to environmental variation—the two scores were highly correlated. The value was 0.93 for the 210 rats of the S_7 generation.

Mating, which of course took place generation by generation within each strain subsequent to the parental generation, which was itself derived from the local albino laboratory stocks, was then carried out on the basis of these scores. Either brother–sister mating or outbreeding—that is, deliberately avoiding such close or indeed other family relationships—was used alternately in successive generations of selection after the S_4 generation. The rationale here was the need to avoid a degree of inbreeding that could prematurely fix the genotypes of possibly less extreme phenotypes than could perhaps be achieved later on in the experiment. This was done by maintaining the maximum variation, which follows from maximizing the opportunities for genetic recombination in a way in which the establishment of substrains, an inevitable consequence of close inbreeding, does not permit. It is well known that bidirectional selection of the kind practiced here can achieve mean scores for later generations, which lie quite outside the range defined by those of the parental strain.

The S_8 generation values for mean alcohol intake during the test period described above showed highly significant differences between the groups with the AA or drinker strain having preference values of 51.2% ± (S.D.) 24.6% for males and 75.3% ± 22.3% for females as opposed to 22.4% ± 16.5% and 29.3% ± 22.7%, respectively, for the ANA or nondrinker strain, thus demonstrating the profound effect that eight generations of disruptive selection pressure of the kind described had wrought in the phenotypes of the two strains concerned. Comparable data for a much later generation (S_{26}), which have recently come to hand (Rusi *et al.,* 1977), yielded the following preference values of 33.5% ± 13.9% (males) and 35.6% ± 16.3% (females) for the AA strain, and of 7.4% ± 7.2% and 8.9% ± 18.1% for the ANA strain, indicative of the sustained and indeed increasing response to selection among the latter.

Much of the rest of Eriksson's (1969*b*) monograph is devoted to studies of the techniques employed in the selection, with relatively little attention to the further study of the strains themselves as thus far developed—perhaps as an outcome of methodological criticism (Myers and Eriksson, 1968) of an earlier report of the first eight generations (Eriksson, 1968*b*) on the grounds that only a single concentration of alcohol was offered as a choice in the preference tests. However, some data were provided which showed quite clearly that one of the responses to selection correlated with the change in alcohol preference and intake in a free-choice situation has been a change in body weight. The AA (drinker) rats were significantly lighter than the nondrinkers (ANA), though both were probably still within normal limits for the rat.

Equally little was given by way of analysis of the genetic and environmental determinants of the striking differences between the strains that were reported, though the results of an experiment in which preference was manipulated by the addition of saccharin or quinine to the alcohol or water, respectively, are of interest. Here the two strains responded in expected ways, that is, by increasing preference, though not always significantly, when either the alcohol solution was sweetened or the water made bitter, or both happened together, and no marked differences were observed between them in these respects. Thus no genotype–environment interaction was observed, as would have been the case if the drinker and nondrinker rats had responded markedly differently to the environmental change imposed by flavor manipulation.

Further reports on this selection experiment (Eriksson, 1968*a,c*) present data at S_9, but, apart from a brief report of a study of the S_{18} generation using an 11.9% (wt./vol.) solution in a choice situation by Eriksson (1972*c*), and the incidental presentation of S_{26} data mentioned above by Rusi *et al.* (1977), the main report has been of the S_{16} generation. Here the figures show (Eriksson, 1971*b*) a sustained and clear-cut response to the further selection with practically no overlap between the two distributions when plotted in terms of the number of calories derived from ethanol consumption as a proportion of the total caloric intake. Inbred strains, started as S_{12}, show a similar differentiation after five generations of such mating. The diurnal rhythm of the alcohol intake of the two strains at S_{15} was studied (Eriksson, 1972*a*) using an automatic recorder that yielded data every hour over a period of 10 days. While the two strains did not differ in their temporal distribution of all fluid intake, blood alcohol levels in the seventeenth-generation animals, when offered a choice between water and 11.9% (wt./vol.) ethanol, varied dramatically. The AA strain was recorded as having at 0400 a mean blood alcohol level of 27 mg % (mg/100 ml) with the probably intoxicating level of 110 being the highest recorded, whereas the ANA gave a mean of 4.2 mg %. Differences in other behavioral characteristics have been reported. At S_{17} the main result found (Eriksson, 1972*b*) was that the ANA strain showed significantly greater ambulation in the open-field test than the AA, while not differing in respect to other measures (for example, defecation) taken therein. Rusi *et al.* (1977) confirmed these findings among saline-injected control groups of rats of the two strains from the S_{26} generation.

Sinclair (1974*b*) studied motivation for alcohol by demonstrating that small numbers of rats of both strains could learn to operate a lever in a Skinner box arranged to deliver 7.9% (wt./vol.) ethanol, and that one AA rat continued to press the bar against a progressively increasing weight loading of it. However, since an unselected Sprague–Dawley control rat performed equally well in this respect, if not better, the significance of this observation is not apparent. No strain difference emerged in a study of the suppression of alcohol intake by the two selected strains occasioned by lithium carbonate given either in the rats' food or by injection (Sinclair, 1974*a*), and since Komura (1974) used only the AA strain in his study of the effect of organic nitrates on ethanol preference, the finding that it was depressed bears little on the subject of strain differences.

However, the main concern of the continuing work on the Alko selected strains has been toward more precisely defining the possible physiological mechanisms underlying the phenotypes differentiated by the manifestly powerful technique of disruptive—that is, two-way—selection employed. Thus, it was shown (Nikander and Pekkanen, 1977) that an injection of 2.5 g/kg of ethanol, given intravenously, differentially affects the motor coordination of rats of the two strains as measured by the tilting plane test discussed in Chapter 2. Performance after 20–40 min was only marginally affected among AA rats, whereas the ANA rats showed performance decrements of nearly 50%, not recovering until after 160 min. Rusi *et al.* (1977) demonstrated that the strains differ in sleep time at S_{20} in response to a standard dose of ethanol. Intubation of 4.0 g/kg into the stomach defined the starting point for the measure of elapsed time to the regaining of the righting reflex. While no difference in blood alcohol levels was reported at that time, the ANA rats slept longer than the AA strain, significantly so among the males.* But no differential sensitivity in open-field ambulation and other activity scores 30 min after a 1.0 g/kg intragastric dose of ethanol was found by these same authors, and it was shown by Forsander and Eriksson (1972) that the rate of ethanol oxidation in response to an injection of 1.5 g/kg of ethanol does not differ between the strains at S_{17}, a finding such as is frequently encountered, as we shall see (Section 9.1), in studies of inbred mouse strains differing in respect to ethanol preference but not its metabolism. It should, however, be noted that data later reported (Eriksson, C. J. P., 1973), which seem to derive from the same experiment, though the sample sizes in three of the four strains by sex groupings were somewhat reduced, did yield a significant interaction of strain with sex. The males did not differ between strains, whereas the females did, the AA ones having the highest of the higher value characteristic for this sex, even though the ANA females also metabolized significantly faster than males of both strains. Similar sampling differences between the two reports apply to the measures of peripheral acetaldehyde—a toxic product to which ethanol is oxidized in the metabolic process by alcohol dehydrogenase—and which, it is hypothesized, may be the basis for unpleasant postingestional effects that could be instrumental in leading to aversion. But both agree in reporting a significantly lower level of acetaldehyde in rats of the AA strain. Forsander and Eriksson (1972) report

---

*The AA strain has also been shown to become less incoordinated after a single dose of ethanol or even *t*-butanol or *n*-propanol. Selection among a heterozygous population of rats for tolerance to ethanol intoxication, using the tilting plane (Chapter 2) test has now begun (Rusi *et al.*, 1977) and the resulting strains named the *a*lcohol *t*olerant (AT) and *a*lcohol *non*-*t*olerant (ANT) strains. In the S_1 generation the significant superiority of the former in resisting performance decrement is again dissociated from blood alcohol levels, which remain similar in the two strains.

other data that support the relevance of this finding to the hypothesis in question: AA rats voluntarily ingest more of a 0.39% (wt./vol.) solution of acetaldehyde itself. Other measures related to alcohol metabolism in which the strains do not differ include their blood sugar curves after ethanol (Forsander and Eriksson, 1972). Measures in which they do differ include the rate of acetaldehyde oxidation (Eriksson, C. J. P., 1973), though confined to within-sex comparisons for technical reasons. The outcome of these biochemical investigations [see also Koivula and Lindros (1975), Koivula *et al.* (1975), and Marselos *et al.* (1975)] leads to the conclusion that "the higher acetaldehyde output during the ethanol oxidation in the ANA strain, as compared with the AA strain, suggests a greater inhibitory influence upon the metabolism of the brain, which could decisively affect behaviour in respect of ethanol preference" (Eriksson, C. J. P., 1973, p. 2291).

Another possible brain mechanism underlying preference was investigated by Ahtee (1972; Ahtee and Eriksson, 1972), using rats from S_{16} and S_{17} generations. Brain serotonin was postulated as causally related since *p*-chlorophenylalanine, a substance which depletes serotonin, has been reported, for example, by Nachman *et al.* (1970) as also reducing alcohol preference in rats. In addition to examining the level in the whole brain—less cerebellum—of serotonin (5-hydroxytryptamine), that of its main metabolite, 5-hydroxyindoleacetic acid, was also investigated to assess the rate of serotonin turnover. Rats never exposed to ethanol showed no significant strain differences, though treatment with probenecid, a 5-hydroxyindoleacetic acid transport inhibitor, increased its level after two hours significantly more in the AA strain than in the ANA strain. A month's exposure to a free choice of 7.9% (wt./vol.) ethanol or water resulted in a significantly higher level of serotonin, but not of its metabolite, in the AA strain than in the ANA strain, though a month on water alone abolished the effect. Forcing alcohol intake on the ANA rats by providing 7.9% ethanol as their only fluid source for a month raised both to levels comparable to those found in the AAs. Further work (Ahtee and Eriksson, 1973) on the regional distribution in the brain of the two amines in rats of the S_{20} generation after six weeks of free choice, showed that the AA rats had significantly higher serotonin levels in the whole brain (as before), in the cortex (which was incidentally significantly heavier in the ANA rats), in the hypothalamus, and in the midbrain plus thalamus. No significant differences in the metabolite were detected, though the AA rats tended to show higher levels of 5-hydroxyindoleacetic acid in most regions examined. Using S_{22} rats, they also showed (Ahtee and Eriksson, 1975) that the total dopamine content of the brain of the AA animals significantly exceeded that of the ANA rats, though the brain noradrenaline did not. While the relation of the preference behavior to brain biochemistry remains unresolved, the authors speculate (Ahtee and Eriksson, 1973) that the high-preference AA strain, whose brain serotonin is so clearly affected by ethanol and whose serotonin metabolism is more susceptible to ethanol, may be responding to pleasurable sensations induced by its ingestion—a truly pharmacodynamic effect—whereas the low-preference strain is merely demonstrating an aversion based on unpalatability of the ethanol solution. Work by Kiianmaa (1975), using the AA strain only, renders this view less likely since he was able to show that the outcome of several different procedures designed to lower brain serotonin was not a lowering of preference in this strain, whereas a similar manipulation of brain noradrenaline did lower preference. Preference was temporarily increased by lesions in the locus coeruleus, which reduced forebrain, especially cortical, noradrenaline stores by as much as 60%. The author suggests that ". . . drinking may be initiated because alcohol is able to increase the release of noradrenaline in the brain and this is reinforcing. It is possible that the increase in alcohol drinking seen in the lesioned rats is their way of increasing the noradrenaline release from the remaining ventral pathways so as to compensate for the loss in the cortical areas" (Kiianmaa, 1975, pp. 81–82). The studies of these selected strains that we have reviewed illustrate, therefore, the two broad hypotheses employed to account for alcohol preference in rodents—pharmacological, that is, postingestional or perceptual, and pre-ingestional—in the variety of explanations advanced to account for the specific findings.

The genetic determination of this preference behavior as evidenced by the Alko strains at the S_{10} generation has been investigated by Eriksson (1969a) using the method of parent–offspring correlational analysis. Prominent in the data is the massive sex difference in preference, already discussed (Chapter 2), which leads to differential effects between the two sexes. Thus the heritability coefficients reported for percentage preference ratios are around 40% if mothers and daughters are included in the calculations, but fall to levels around 10% if fathers or sons are involved. This led Eriksson to invoke sex linkage as a possible explanation of these differences, supporting this suggestion with results briefly reported earlier (Eriksson, 1968b) and derived from first and second filial crosses, apparently using the AA and ANA strains at S_7 as the parental strains for this Mendelian analysis. But the details given are insufficient to evaluate the outcome and the methodology used is probably insufficiently precise to establish such unusual genetical architecture for a behavioral trait, so that confirmation is required before such a claim can be entertained.

This extensive research effort has given rise to behavioral strains of considerable interest which, in turn, have prompted a series of investigations employing them. They are summarized for convenience in Table II.

TABLE II

Psychopharmacological Selection: The Alko Rat Strains

Reference	Generation	Measure	Outcome	Remarks
Eriksson (1972a)	S_{15}	Automatic hourly fluid intake Preference test	No significant (n.s.) difference AA Blood alcohol level significantly higher	
Eriksson (1972b)	S_{17}	Open-field test	ANA greater ambulation, n.s. difference defecation	
Sinclair (1974a)	?	Lithium carbonate suppression of alcohol ingestion	n.s. difference	
Sinclair (1974b)	?	Operant lever pressing for ethanol	One AA pressed against increasing lever weight	Unselected control pressed equally well
Komura (1974)	?	Organic nitrates on alcohol ingestion	Reduced ingestion	AA only
Forsander and Eriksson (1972)	S_{17}	Metabolism, ethanol oxidation after injection	n.s. difference in postethanol blood sugar, or ethanol oxidation	Similar findings in mice
		Peripheral acetaldehyde	AA lower	
Eriksson, C.J.P. (1973)	S_{17}	As Forsander and Eriksson (1972)	Significant interaction strain × sex AA females faster oxidation AA lower acetaldehyde Difference in acetaldehyde oxidation	Acetaldehyde (a toxic metabolite of ethanol) postulated as instrumental to aversion

Reference		Method	Result	Comment
Ahtee (1972)	S_{16}–S_{17}	Whole-brain serotonin	n.s. difference in naïve rats	Serotonin preference relations since serotonin depletor also reduces preference
Ahtee and Eriksson (1972)		Whole-brain assay of serotonin metabolite (5-hydroxyindole-acetic acid)	Higher serotonin (not metabolite) in AA exposure to ethanol	
Ahtee and Eriksson (1973)	S_{20}	Whole-brain serotonin Regional serotonin	AA higher AA higher n.s. difference in metabolite	
Ahtee and Eriksson (1975)	S_{22}	Whole-brain dopamine Whole-brain noradrenaline	AA higher n.s. difference	
Kiianmaa (1975)	?	Preference after serotonin reduction Preference after brain noradrenaline manipulation	No change Reduced	Argues against ANA response as simple alcohol aversion
Eriksson (1969a)	S_{10}	Parent–offspring correlation analysis	Preference heritabilities: 10%, males; 40%, females	Sex linkage?
Nikander and Pekkanen (1977)	?	Tilting plane after ethanol	ANA performance disrupted	
Rusi et al. (1977)	S_{20} S_{26}	Sleep time after ethanol Blood alcohol Open-field test	ANA (males only) longer n.s. difference ANA greater ambulation	Confirms Eriksson (1972b)

This Finnish selection experiment amply confirmed the findings of a previous, less extensive one, in which selection for alcohol preference was also practiced in rats, the reports on which are included in Table III. Mardones *et al.* (1950) showed that even one generation of selection, though in a positive direction only, could have some effect on mean alcohol preference, and a second report (Mardones *et al.*, 1953) yielded a form of heritability coefficient of the order of 40%. But this breeding program was not a selection experiment in the usual sense, even though the work was extended to include a low-preference strain, as a later report by Mardones (1960) makes clear. In it he published pedigrees for many generations (16 in the case of the high-preference strain, and 14 in the case of the low), which suggest that while some selection pressure was certainly exerted, the main purpose was to inbreed with descendants of certain pairs of individuals. As we have seen, this is not the best breeding system to combine with genetical selection. Segovia-Riquelme *et al.* (1971) carried the account further with outline pedigrees to the S_{34} generation of the low-preference strain, now designated the UCh-A, and the S_{29} generation of the high-preference strain (UCh-B). Crossing the two strains yielded a sizable F_1 of 53 rats, whose mean daily intake value fell rather squarely between the values quoted for the parents. The generation from which they were drawn was not given, though S_{37} of the A (low–preference) strain and S_{31} of the B (high–preference) appear to have been reached. The only other attempt at a genetical analysis is a somewhat speculative interpretation of phenotypic distributions within the two strains in terms of major genes (Mardones, 1968), which is rendered less likely by the intermediate F_1 value referred to above. Further work, in one case (Segovia-Riquelme *et al.*, 1962) apparently using these strains, and in another (Segovia-Riquelme *et al.*, 1964) definitely, yielded no evidence of differences between them in the rate of metabolism of injected alcohol, but showed both glucose and gluconate metabolism to be higher in the high-preference strain. A further selection experiment for this phenotype, this time in mice, was briefly reported by Anderson and McClearn (1975). Five generations of bidirectional selection from a parental population specially bred to be heterogeneous produced striking differences between the two strains in their alcohol–preference scores after 24 hr of water deprivation. This study repeated and extended an earlier one (Rodgers and McClearn, 1962*a*) in which data from one generation only were reported (see Table III).

If the alcohol preference of laboratory animals presents problems of definition perhaps too behavioral and insufficiently pharmacological for the genetics of it to fall within the purview of this monograph (see page 7, footnote), then the opposite may perhaps be argued in relation to studies in which phenotypes relating to toxicity (especially as seen in convulsivity and mortality), anesthesia, sedation, and the like are investigated. However, an important bidirectional selection for sleep time in mice in response to a dose of 3.4 mg/kg of ethyl alcohol (McClearn and Kakihana, 1973) merits attention since, even though briefly reported, it had achieved S_{14} animals with practically no overlap in the distributions of the two strains. By the S_{18} generation no overlap whatsoever is reported (Sanders, 1976), the average sleep times being 2.3 hr for the *long sleep* (LS) strain and 11 min for the *short sleepers* (SS), though now in response to a hypnotic dose of 4.1 g/kg ethanol. McClearn (1973) also presents details of the first five generations of selection. Realized heritability, that is, the ratio of the response to selection to the amount of selection pressure exerted by the choice of parents in each generation up to S_5, is reported as 18%.

Furthermore, these selected long- and short-sleep strains have already been studied in other investigations, the results of some of which are indicative of a genotype–environment interaction. An investigation of their alcohol preference, briefly reported by Fuller and Church (1977), hints at the complexity of causal mechanisms operating, since the LS strain showed a clearly lower preference than the SS mice. This difference could, however, be enhanced by previous experience of drinking alcohol. Chan (1976), on the other hand, mentions unpublished data which suggest that both strains exhibit low alcohol preference, and presents results, derived from males of the S_{18} generation, in which the response to an intraperitoneal injection of 4 g/kg ethanol was studied 30 and 90 min later for its effect on the neurotransmitter γ-aminobutyric acid (GABA) content of the brain. Various regions were assayed, but no significant differences were found beyond a generally significant increase due to ethanol as compared with saline controls; nor were differences between the strains the major effect, GABA levels being similar in the two strains both before and after treatment. While Heston *et al.* (1973, 1974) showed, and Siemens and Chan (1975) confirmed, that the strains did not differ in respect of their hepatic metabolism of alcohol—the difference probably residing in the specific sensitivity of the LS strain to the depressant effects of alcohols, especially ethanol, on the central nervous sytem—others have briefly reported (Collins and Deitrich, 1973) that the rate of turnover of another neurotransmitter in the brain (dopamine) was differentially affected by injected alcohol, the SS strain being less affected than the LS strain. A reverse pattern of effects was detected for the other neuroamine studied, norepinephrine. Kakihana (1976) demonstrated that the LS strain at the S_{16} generation showed a significantly higher corticosterone response in both sexes to injected alcohol, though no difference in responses to histamine (females only) or to foot shock were found. The time course of the development of the response was shown to be parallel in the two strains, though the interpretation of

TABLE III
Other Psychopharmacological Selections Relating to Alcohol

Reference	Method	Measure	Strain/Generation	Outcome	Remarks
Mardones et al. (1950, 1953)	One-way selection	Alcohol preference	S_{16}	Mean preference affected positively	
Mardones (1960)	Rats inbred within descendants of extreme pairs				Suboptimal procedure
Segovia-Riquelme et al. (1971)	F_1 cross	Alcohol preference	UCh-A (low) UCh-B (high) /S_{37}	Preference values mid-parental	Result argues against major gene hypothesis (Mardones, 1968)
Segovia-Riquelme et al. (1962, 1964)	Alcohol injection	Metabolism	UCh-A, UCh-B	n.s. difference but UCh-B higher glucose and gluconate metabolism	
Anderson and Mc-Clearn (1975)	Bidirectional selection/mice	Alcohol preference	S_5	Striking strain difference after water deprivation	Extension of Rodgers and McClearn (1962a)
McClearn and Kakihana (1973)	Bidirectional selection/mice	Sleep time after ethanol	SS (short) LS (long)	Realized heritability 18% at S_5	
Sanders (1976)	Bidirectional selection/mice	Alcohol preferences	SS, LS/S_{18}	No overlap in distributions	
Fuller and Church (1977)		Alcohol preference	SS, LS	LS lower; previous alcohol enhances difference	Genotype-environment interaction?
Heston et al. (1973, 1974)		Alcohol metabolism	SS, LS	n.s. difference	Confirmed by Siemens and Chan (1975)
Collins and Deitrich (1973)	Alcohol injection	Dopamine turnover Norepinephrine turnover	SS, LS	SS less affected LS less affected	
Erwin et al. (1976)	Injections of ethanol, methanol, n-butanol	Sleep time	SS, LS/S_{14}	Strain difference	

Reference	Treatment	Measure	Strains	Result	Comments
Chan (1976)	Injections of paraldehyde, pentobarbital, chloral hydrate trichloroethanol / Injection of t-butanol / Etherization	Righting reflexes	SS, LS/S_{18}	Strain difference / No strain difference / Both strains low	
	Ethanol injected	Alcohol preference	?	n.s. difference	
Kakihana (1976)		Brain GABA content 30/90 min later	SS, LS/S_{16} males	LS higher	SS responded more to injection *per se* / SS larger adrenals
	Alcohol injection / Histamine injection / Foot shock	Corticosterone response	SS, LS/S_{16}	LS higher / n.s. difference / n.s. difference	
Goldstein and Kakihana (1975)	Alcohol fuming	Withdrawal reaction	SS, LS/S_{17}	SS more susceptible	
Kakihana and Moore (1977)	Alcohol injection / Saline injection	Rectal temperature	SS, LS	SS lower / SS higher	n.s. differences to pentrylene, tetrazol, chloroform, or paraldehyde
Baer and Crumpacker (1975)	Pre- and postnatal alcohol exposure, F_1 cross	Alcohol preference	SS, LS	Prenatal treatment facilitated	
Sanders (1976)	Alcohol and pentobarbital injections	Open-field test	SS, LS/S_{18}	Ambulation increased significantly more in SS	
Church et al. (1976)	Coordination after alcohol injection	Rotating rod	SS, LS	n.s. difference	Confirmed by Church (1977)
	Salsolinol injection	Sleep time	SS, LS	LS longer	Relationship between salsolinol and ethanol metabolites
Vander Vliet and Crumpacker (1976)	F_1 cross	Response to ethanol and butanol	SS, LS	No maternal effect	Potence differences for these two alcohols
Goldstein (1973)	Bidirectional selection after alcohol fuming/mice	Withdrawal reactions	S_2	Significant difference seizure scores	Breeding after fuming may constitute artifact

these data is complicated by a greater response in the SS strain to the injection procedure as such, as demonstrated by the values for the saline control animals. This finding is supported by the data presented on their significantly larger adrenal gland weights and suggestive of a greater pituitary–adrenal sensitivity in this strain in contrast to the specific CNS sensitivity to alcohol in the LS mice, noted above. Goldstein and Kakihana (1975) showed that at the S_{17} generation the SS mice were similarly more susceptible to withdrawal reactions than the LS mice after the inhalation of alcohol vapor. This technique of fuming was combined with injections of pyrazole designed to prevent the oxidation of alcohol and hence to maintain blood concentrations as high as possible for three days. The actual mean values were 172 and 164 mg/100 ml for SS and LS groups, respectively. Physical dependence on alcohol can now be observed in that convulsions in response to handling develop within a few hours after withdrawal, persisting at a relatively high level of expression up to 18 hr in the SS strain, whereas the LS animals show milder reactions up to 10 hr only. Similarly, it was the SS strain that showed (Kakihana and Moore, 1977) greater hypothermic effects on rectal temperature in response to an injection of 2.0 g/kg of ethanol as well as a greater hyperthermia to saline injections. That no further strain interactions were detected in response to injections of the convulsants pentylenetetrazol, chloroform, and paraldehyde was informally reported by Erwin, Heston, McClearn, and Deitrich (in Kakihana, 1976; Sanders, 1976), and confirmed in respect to paraldehyde (1.0 g/kg) by Erwin *et al.* (1976). In this study it was also shown that pentobarbital (0.60 g/kg), chloral hydrate (0.45 g/kg), and trichloroethanol (0.225 g/kg) were similarly without significant differential effect on the sleep times of the S_{14} generation of the two strains, who now responded, however, with the usual massive differences in sleep time in response to 3.75 g/kg of ethanol. The values were 2.6 hr for the LS animals and 6 min for the SS animals. These workers likewise confirmed the group's previous report (Heston *et al.*, 1973) that other alcohols, specifically methanol (4.5 g/kg) and *n*-butanol (0.567 g/kg), yield similarly striking differences in sleep time. With loss of righting reflexes as the measure, the range of agents studied was extended using S_{18} subjects to include ether, which, like the other nonalcohol central nervous system depressants tested, showed little strain difference, and *t*-butanol, which resembled the other alcohols in demonstrating once again the marked sensitivity of the LS strain mice. Siemens' and Chan's brief report (1975), while indicating a differential loss of righting reflexes between the strains in response to pentobarbital (0.50 g/kg)—in contradistinction to the findings reported above—yet again confirmed by other measures the apparent equisensitivity of the strains to the barbiturate as opposed to their response to ethanol.

Erwin *et al.* (1976) confirmed the deduction from such findings that since no differences in alcohol metabolism between the two strains had been detected (as noted earlier), yet the LS mice sleep so much longer, they must therefore awaken with much lower blood alcohol levels. Of greater importance, however, was the demonstration that the strains do not vary significantly in the toxicity of alcohol, the LD_{50} being 4.5 (LS) and 4.8 g/kg (SS).

Equally, Baer and Crumpacker (1975), in an interesting study of the effects of pre- and postnatal exposure to alcohol in offspring of the two strains at the S_{15} generation, showed that the prenatal treatment had merely overall facilitatory effects on preference for alcohol. The findings of MacInnes and Damjanovich (1973) seemed to point to the existence of enzyme systems other than the alcohol dehydrogenase pathway in the metabolism of ethanol. Interactions were, however, evident in the long- and short-sleep strains' reaction at the S_{18} generation to low doses of ethanol (1.4, 1.8, and 2.0 g/kg) as measured in the open-field test, in which the ambulatory activity of the mice was increased in both strains, as compared with saline controls, but significantly more in the SS strain (Sanders, 1976). However, when their coordination was tested by their ability to remain on a rod rotating at progressively increasing speeds, ethanol showed an equally disruptive effect. These observations were confirmed by Church (1977), though using a slightly different range of doses (1.0–2.0 g/kg) and tests. Sanders (1976) also reports that pentobarbital in five doses from 8 to 28 mg/kg had a similar though less pronounced effect on open-field ambulation. Church *et al.* (1976) sought to investigate directly the effect on these two selected strains of a tetrahydroisoquinoline compound, salsolinol. This is a condensation product from the reaction of dopamine with acetaldehyde, detectable in the rat brain during acute exposure to ethanol. Direct injection of salsolinol into the brain (240 μg into the cisterna cerebromedullaris) gave significantly longer sleep times in the LS strain than in the SS strain, and a graduated series of smaller doses (10, 20, 30, and 40 μg) produced a roughly parallel decrease in the measured activity of both strains. The possibility of a genetical relationship of salsolinol to biochemical activities initiated by ethanol is strengthened by the observation that injected acetaldehyde also produces a drug–strain interaction in the shape of significant differences in sleep time between the selected strains, but, as the authors point out, it may be that these differences are merely correlated responses to the selection procedure for ethanol sleep times. Finally, in a brief report of an important investigation involving crossbreeding these selected strains, Vander Vliet and Crumpacker (1976) present data showing that there is no maternal effect in the F_1 response to either ethanol or butanol but that the potence (apparent dominance)

(Chapter 6) differs for the two alcohols used. The already considerable amount of work employing these two interesting strains is summarized in Table III. It provides further evidence of the value of selection studies in this field. Moreover, as Erwin *et al.* (1976) point out, it is now possible to be reasonably secure in characterizing the response to drugs that the selection process has been operating upon. It is not a general sensitivity to depressants of the central nervous system since the nonalcohols do not differentiate the strains. "This observation is somewhat surprising since all the tested compounds (pentobarbital, ether, chloral hydrate, and paraldehyde) are at least additive with ethanol in their effects on the CNS. In particular, ether, chloral hydrate, and paraldehyde have long been thought to possess a similar if not identical mechanism to that of ethanol. These results permit a conclusion that the mechanism of these compounds all differ in some respect from that of ethanol even though the final common result is the same" (Erwin *et al.*, 1976, p. 682). Similarly, they argue that, because the sensitivity to other alcohols tested resembles that for ethanol (the one used for producing the original selection pressure in creating the strains) despite the differing metabolic routes, then a brain sensitivity to alcohols in general has been achieved. This argument is thus based on correlated responses to selection, but the difference in potence for two of the alcohols noted above suggests that the genetic architecture for the different alcohols may not be identical. However, what is clear is that the genetic architecture(s) governing the sensitivity to alcohols must be different for the sleep phenotype from that governing ethanol toxicity since the strains do not differ in respect of the overdosage required to produce death. In this way, the complexity of the interaction of drug and genetic background is coming to be revealed by these studies of McClearn and his group.

The same can hardly be claimed for yet another selection study (Riley *et al.*, 1976) for sleep time in response to injected alcohol, this time in rats. Responding to what they perceive as the deficiencies of previous psychogenetical work in providing an animal analog for human alcoholism, they commenced a bidirectional selection study for the decrement in activity as measured in activity platforms during 15–30 min after an intraperitoneal injection of 1.5 g/kg of alcohol (presumably ethanol). The parental population was derived from a mixture of Sprague–Dawley albinos and Long–Evans hooded rats. While the husbandry of the rats was carefully controlled, as is requisite in a selective breeding study, various modifications had been made in the test procedure before the S_5 generation and, more importantly, in the methods by which parents for successive generations had been made in the test procedure before the S_5 generation and, responses achieved after eight generations of selection—there being greater increase in response in the *m*ost *a*ffected (MA) strain than in the practically nonexistent response of the rats bred for minimal effect of alcohol, the *l*east *a*ffected (LA) strain—was overcome at the S_9 generation by a change in selection policy. A switch to the more appropriate technique of selecting extreme phenotypes for breeding, irrespective of familial relationships, doubtless occasioned the marked improvement in the values for the LA strain, yielding mean values for the ratios of decrease in activity after alcohol to about 90% reduction for the MA strain as opposed to nearly 50% for LA rats. Further details regarding the use of these strains in other experimentation can be found in Riley *et al.* (1977) and Worsham *et al.* (1977).

Comparable reservations regarding behavioral relevance to those reviewed above in respect to the relationship of sleep time to alcohol injection also apply to a study by Goldstein (1973, noted in Table III) in which two generations of bidirectional selection were used for investigating hereditary influences on withdrawal reactions after fuming with alcohol vapor in the manner described above. Selective breeding from among the parental population of Swiss albino mice showed an apparent pronounced effect on the subsequent seizure scores, but insufficient details of the measures taken to maintain that constancy of environment necessary for the unequivocal demonstration of a hereditary effect are given for the reader to be complacent on this score. In particular, it would appear that the mice were bred in the selected generations *after* fuming. Without invoking Lamarckian hypotheses it might be possible to speculate that the blood chemistry of the susceptible parents had been so radically altered that the prenatal environment of their offspring could have been directly modified to allow a constitutional effect to be mediated in this way, rather than by differences in genetic mechanisms. However, it could be argued that this is so unlikely a possibility that it is unnecessary to employ either of the alternative techniques required to control for it, namely, splitting litters in each generation and breeding from that portion only which had not been fumed, or routinely breeding from *all* subjects in the experiment before fuming, and discarding from it those offspring of parents who proved not to have extreme scores.

Other psychopharmacological selection work has been concerned with morphine. Nichols (1962, 1964; Nichols and Hsiao, 1967) has reported on two selections for behavior in Sprague–Dawley rats which is claimed to be an analog of human dependence. Rats normally reject a morphine solution in favor of water in a free-choice situation. However after a regimen comprising three periods during which, first, morphine hydrochloride is injected daily for 17 days, followed by, second, a 30-day period involving a series of trials in which morphine consumption is forced by water deprivation on the previous day, and followed by, third, a period during which no morphine is given for 14 days during which physiological functioning normalizes, some rats now voluntarily take larger amounts of an aqueous solution of morphine (0.5 mg/ml water) than they took before such a regimen. In the first experiment (Nichols, 1962), interbreeding those rats which showed varying degrees of such a preference, that is, one generation of selection, yielded offspring resembling their parents in this respect, and possible artifacts such as difference in taste threshold and body weight were excluded. Mention was also made of two experiments in which high- and low-scoring groups were compared with respect to their emotional reactivity, as observed in Hall's open-field test (Hall, 1934; Broadhurst, 1960), with results which, while too briefly reported to evaluate adequately, were suggestive of no difference. In passing, we may note that this question can be posed in the opposite sense: Would there then have been a correlated response in preference if selection had been for extremes of emotionality? Experimentation to be discussed later has provided some answer to this question, at least with respect to alcohol preference, a phenotype also studied in these strains in the manner discussed below.

Postnatal maternal effects were later examined (Nichols, 1964) on the presumably now established "addiction-prone" and "-resistant" strains by the standard technique of crossfostering offspring to be reared by foster mothers of the opposing strain. There were persisting differences, up to 42 days after forced intake, between their morphine preferences, despite this important macroenvironmental variation, so that, irrespective of fostering, the high-preference rats drank about double the amount of morphine drunk by the low-preference ones. These findings confirm that the strain differences have a strong heritable component. It should, however, be noted that this test does not exclude another possible maternal effect—the prenatal one of the influence of strain differences in maternal environment *in utero*, postconception but preparturition. Reciprocal breeding between established strains is the appropriate technique for pursuing this possibility (Broadhurst, 1961). See Section 9.1 for further discussion of this point.

Selection to the S_3 generation was reported in a new experiment (Nichols and Hsiao, 1967) in which a 25% selection pressure was exerted to provide the parents for each succeeding generation, a clear bidirectional effect being reported, with the high-preference line diverging significantly from the low by the third generation. Interestingly, the preference scores of the high-preference animals, before the induction of the morphine-directed behavior, show both extreme aversion initially and no sign of change in successive generations. Their scores show more aversion than is demonstrated by the low-preference strain even at the S_3 generation. These observations confirm that the high-preference phenotype is the outcome of the environmental manipulation, and that the selection practiced has not resulted in a strain spontaneously morphine-oriented without training. This is not, of course, to minimize the importance selection has had in determining the susceptibility (or otherwise) of genotypes to such training. On the other hand, a preference test for 7.9% (wt./vol.) alcohol yielded a significant difference in the direction of a positively correlated response to both drugs, but only after the regimen imposed on the naïve females from the two strains had been made somewhat more rigorous. It should be noted that this is a different situation from the alcohol-preference tests previously discussed, in which only a relatively short period of preliminary exposure to the drug was used.

Mention should be made of work by Gut and Becker (1975) on hexobarbital sleep time in rats, their report of which includes data on five generations of bidirectional group selection from a Wistar parental strain and one generation from a Sprague–Dawley group. The phenotype was defined as the mean of two or three measurements of the time between the loss and the recovery of the righting reflex after an injection (i.p.) of hexobarbital sodium, the dose being varied for strain and for sex, presumably to take approximate account of body weight differences. Thus the males of both strains received 150 mg/kg, but Wistar females 100 mg/kg and Sprague–Dawley animals 75 mg/kg. One generation of selection among the latter strain not surprisingly showed little effect on the phenotype, but by the S_5 generation in the former, differences were observed, though they were more striking in the long-sleep strain, being over twice the parental values among males and approaching that ratio among females, suggesting some asymmetry in the response to the selection pressure exerted. Study of young subjects from the S_4 generation showed a fairly marked increase in sleep time between four and eight weeks of age, and at S_5 various measures of liver metabolism were shown to be accelerated in the short-sleep strain. The liver size comparison, on the other hand, favored the long-sleep strain. No other behavioral measures were reported, and the volume of work on these selected strains does not as yet rival that using the mouse strains developed using a similar phenotype (sleep time), though in response to alcohol, as discussed above. Table IV presents a summary of the studies reviewed.

The genetical conclusions, which can be drawn from all the psychopharmacological selection experiments described, are constrained not only by the inherent limitations of the method but also by the failure to push it to its possible limits. Thus, for example, few calculations of the realized heritability of the phenotypes under selection have been presented except by McClearn and Kakihana (1973), nor have possible asymmetries in the progress of selection in the different directions been adequately documented.

TABLE IV

Further Psychopharmacological Selections

Reference	Method	Measure	Generation	Outcome	Remarks
Nichols and Hsiao (1967) Nichols (1962, 1964)	Bidirection selection, rats habituated to morphine	Morphine preference	S_1	Selection already effective	Taste threshold and body-weight artifacts excluded?
	Cross-fostering offspring	Morphine preference	?	Maternal effects n.s.	No *prenatal* control
Nichols and Hsiao (1967)	New bidirection selection, rats habituated to morphine	Morphine preference	S_3	Clear bidirectional effect. High-preference strain shows aversion before habituation	No spontaneous morphine preference
Gut and Becker (1975)	Bidirectional selection, rats after hexobarbital sodium	Sleep time	S_5	Differences found, asymmetry toward LS	
		Liver metabolism		Accelerated in SS	
		Liver size		Larger in LS	
Rusi *et al.* (1977)	Bidirectional selection after intragastric ethanol	Tilting plane	AT, ANT/S_1	ANT more susceptible	
		Blood alcohol		n.s. difference	
Riley *et al.* (1976)	Bidirectional selection after intraperitoneal alcohol injection, rats	Activity platform	MA, LA/ S_8-S_9	n.s. difference	

These and other questions (Falconer, 1960) can be approached in the analysis of the outcome of selection, with consequent illumination of the genetic mechanisms involved. It remains for future work to attempt this. It may be that further reports of progress toward the usual criterion of twenty generations of selection for the establishment of uniform strains will carry these matters further, but for the moment all that can be claimed for the material reviewed is that it shows a *prima facie* case for a considerable degree of genetic involvement in the determination of the psychopharmacological phenotypes studied. Selection was in each case to a large degree successful and some, but by no means all, of the more obvious environmental artifacts that could perturb this conclusion have been excluded as causal. Some indications of correlated response to the selections practiced strengthen this appraisal.

Chapter 4

Other Selections

Far more abundant use has been made in psychopharmacology of strains of rats (especially), which were created by selective breeding but for some phenotype, usually a behavioral one, other than the psychopharmacological ones we have hitherto been considering. Usually such selections have been made bidirectionally and hence their use in this connection constitutes a special case of the more general approach to psychogenetics via the study of strain differences. Mention has already been made (see Chapter 3) of the Tyron rat strains, the *maze-b*right and -*d*ull (TMB and TMD), and consideration of contributions based on their use is given pride of place.

In addition to their intrinsic value in psychogenetics, partly because of their early foundation in America in the 1920s—a time when interest in hereditary determinants of behavior was at a low ebb—and their survival through World War II, and partly because of the frequency with which they are cited as evidence in the intermittently recurring controversies over the determinants of human intelligence, the Tryon strains and the selection experiments that gave rise to them are exceedingly widely known. Only a brief description of the foundation of these strains is therefore necessary. Tryon's work began in 1927 using an automatic 17-unit maze and he selectively bred for 22 generations (Tryon, 1931, 1940, 1942). He started with a parental group heterogeneous for coat color but by the S_{22} generation the maze-bright strain, that is the one making fewer errors in the maze learning, was mostly brown and the maze-dull strain, black. Selection was abandoned during World War II, but fortunately the stocks were maintained as two distinct strains without outbreeding, though the number of generations they passed through is not known.

Starting from the late 1950s, a considerable body of work employing these strains has been reported, of which the pharmacological side we are to explore—summarized in Table V—is only a part. Earlier work was surveyed by Rosenzweig (1964); and later work, much of which was concentrated in the psychopharmacological field and was related to the consolidation of learning, has been reviewed by McGaugh (1973; McGaugh and Herz, 1972) from that point of view. Some of these early studies were also superior to those that came later, using other selected strains, both in terms of the quality of the work, insofar as that can be judged from published reports, and, as is especially relevant to the present review, from the possibility they afforded of genetical analysis of a drug phenotype. This situation arose because several studies employed the TMB and TMD strains as parental generations and crossed them to provide an F_1 generation or first filial cross, which was also tested in the context of the same experiment, thus providing the minimum breeding design for the detection of genetic effects. The point here is that differences between strains as such, even when inbred, are only presumptive evidence that genetic differences underlie the phenotypic differences observed. First the possibility of environmental artifacts must be excluded and, even if that can be done satisfactorily, no analysis of the putative genetic variables is possible without the involvement of meiosis and the processes of chromosomal rearrangement therein implied. In a word, the genetic process itself, that is, the breeding of another generation at least, must be involved as an independent variable in order that its nature may be explored. Selection, of course, achieves this by successive, and often many, generations of assortative mating based on matching phenotypic extremes. The end result of this process is that some degree of genetical analysis is possible, though it has as yet not been much applied in psychopharmacology, as we have seen. The more usual and generally more efficient genetic approach (Jinks and Broadhurst, 1974) is by breeding from two or more inbred parental strains their first and second filial crosses (F_1 and F_2, respectively) and backcrosses, preferably reciprocally in each case in order to test for the presence of prenatal maternal effects of the kind already mentioned.

Two investigations employing the TMB and TMD strains of rats can be used to exemplify this approach, albeit only on a limited scale. McGaugh and his associates have used the minimum breeding design of parental strains, the two Tryon strains in this case, and the F_1 cross between them to study the effect on learning and memory of a strychnine-like stimulant, diphenyl diazadamantan, depending on when the same dose (1 mg/kg) was injected, either 10 min before (McGaugh *et al.*, 1961) or 1 min after (McGaugh *et al.*, 1962a), and how the daily training in a Lashley III maze

TABLE V

Pharmacology and Psychogenetic Selection: The Tryon Rat Strains

Reference	Treatment	Measure	Outcome	Remarks
McGaugh et al. (1961)	Diphenyl diazadamantan 10 min before	Lashley III maze: massed trials	Significant drug–strain interaction	F₁ included: Analysis could be carried further
McGaugh et al.(1962a)	Diphenyl diazadamantan 1 min after	Lashley III maze: spaced trials	Significant drug–strain interaction	
McGaugh and Petrinovich (1959)	Strychnine sulfate	Lashley III maze	Learning facilitated	F₁ only: Partially replicated, Long–Evans hooded rats (Petrinovich, 1967)
McGaugh (1961)	Strychnine, two doses	14-unit T-maze	Low dose facilitated learning, high dose disrupted	F₁, only
Breen and McGaugh (1961)	Picrotoxin, increasing doses	14-unit T-maze	Greater (but n.s.) facilitation and retention in TMDs	
McGaugh and Thomson (1962)	Strychnine	Visual discrimination learning	Same facilitatory effect as in maze learning	
Petrinovich (1963)	Strychnine	Visual discrimination learning	n.s. difference	Facilitation of higher dosage confirmed
Ross (1964)	Strychnine immediately or 1 hr after	14-unit maze	TMD facilitated immediately, TMB at 1 hr	
Westbrook and McGaugh (1964)	Diphenyl diazadamantan immediately after	6-unit maze	Learning facilitated	
Burt (1962)	Picrotoxin, increasing doses	Seizure threshold	TMD more resistant but lower fatality threshold	
Stratton and Petrinovich (1963)	Physostigmine 2 min after	Lashley III maze	Learning facilitated, dose-response curve interacted with strain	
Powell et al. (1967)	Amobarbital 20 min before	Escape avoidance conditioning	Significant dose-strain interaction	
Russell and Stern (1973)	Ethanol	Acceptance of daily increase	TMB higher final concentration	Contrasting sex
Drewek and Broadhurst (1978)	Alcohol preference	Six different concentrations	TMB higher	Sex differences
	Alcohol injection	Sleep time	n.s. difference	

for a food reward was given, being either massed in the first experiment or spaced in the second.*

Thus, in each case we have three strains, measured under two conditions, control injection and drugged, so that the drug response can be evaluated as a phenotype in its own right. In each case the strain × treatment term in the analysis of variance of mean errors was significant and biometrical analysis should allow us to carry the matter somewhat further. Unfortunately the data from the two experiments are not exactly comparable, since a *pre*injection was combined with *massed* trials in the first and a *post*injection with *spaced* training in the second experiment and, moreover, the reported number of learning trials varied. Only an impressionistic interpretation of the results shown in Figure 1 can therefore be attempted, and from it one can do little more than say that it seems that the drug is interacting with genotype rather differently in the two cases. In the first experiment (prior injection, massed trials) the evident genetic differences, with the parental strains showing the expected extreme phenotypic values and the filial cross (F_1) occupying an intermediate position between them, are largely obliterated by the drug, which selectively affects the groups by raising the TMB rats' error score and lowering (that is, improving) quite markedly that of the TMDs. The postinjection combined with spaced training, on the other hand, did little for the performance of the dull strain, but clearly improved that of both the brights and the F_1—a process that accentuated the differences between them not especially evident in the control groups, injected after training with only the citrate buffer solution used as a placebo.

Further work on the TMB and TMD strains and crosses between them has also been reported, largely by McGaugh's group, but not in such a way as to enable pharmacogenetic analysis of the kind referred to. McGaugh and Petrinovich (1959) reported one experiment in which only the F_1 cross was injected with strychnine sulfate, which facilitated their learning of a Lashley III maze, a study replicated later (Petrinovich, 1967) with only partial success, probably due to the use of a different strain of rats (Long-Evans hooded). McGaugh (1961) also restricted himself to the F_1 cross between the Tryons as subjects in a study employing strychnine sulfate in two dosages in addition to a placebo before single daily trials in a 14-unit T-maze. As compared to the group receiving a placebo the low-dosage group made fewer errors, whereas the high dose proved disruptive in that more errors were made.

*In the second case, the published paper reports the values for the TMB and TMD strains only; those for the F_1 cross were kindly made available to me by Professor McGaugh (personal communications, 1960, 1975).

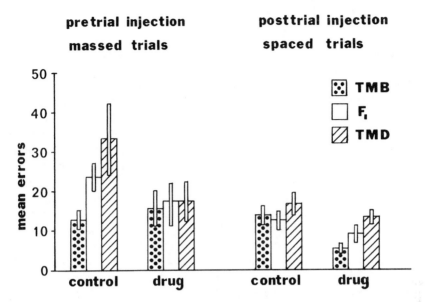

Fig. 1. Drug–strain interactions in response to diphenyl-diazadamantan in the rat. The bar diagrams on the left show the mean and one standard deviation (centered on the mean) of the number of errors made in 14 trials on four successive days in a four-unit maze for a food reward; that is, relatively massed trials were used and 1.0 mg/kg diphenyl-diazadamantan was injected intraperitoneally 10 min before the first of the daily trials. Data are from McGaugh *et al.* (1961), redrawn from Broadhurst (1964). The bar diagrams on the right show data in the same form for the same measure but for errors recorded on days 2–5 on which a single trial was immediately followed by diphenyl-diazadamantan. Data from McGaugh *et al.* (1962*a* and personal communication).

On the other hand, several studies used the parental strains without any representatives of crosses between them: Thus, Breen and McGaugh (1961) found that increasing doses of picrotoxin, a medullary stimulant, given after trials in the same maze facilitated learning and retention in the TMDs more than in the TMBs, though the interaction did not attain significance, and McGaugh and Thomson (1962) showed that strychnine had the same facilitatory effect on visual discrimination learning in the strains as on maze learning when administered before training. Petrinovich (1963) confirmed that strychnine facilitated discrimination learning using the higher dosage, which McGaugh (1961) had found disruptive. No strain difference in response to the drug was detected. Ross (1964), however, in a preliminary report of an experiment in which strychnine (dose not stated) was given either immediately after maze learning trials or one hour later, found a strain difference in response. The TMB rats were facilitated at the longer interval and not at the shorter, whereas with the TMDs the reverse was obtained.

The effect of diphenyl-diazadamantan on the latent learning of a 6-unit maze was investigated in the two strains in the usual manner, that is, by running some rats in it with food-rewarded trials and others first unrewarded and later rewarded. In each case, the drug was injected immediately after daily trials (Westbrook and McGaugh, 1964). The analysis of the results showed that the drug had a facilitatory effect on learning, but while some strain differences were detected, there was no drug–strain interaction. Stratton and Petrinovich (1963) compared the strains in respect to their response to physostigmine salicylate, which affects the cholinergic system in the brain by interfering with the action of the enzyme, acetylcholinesterase, in inactivating acetylcholine. Posttrial injections in a range of doses from 0.25 to 1.0 mg/kg, administered 2 min after daily training for a food reward in a Lashley III maze gave a clear indication that performance, in terms of trials to criterion, was enhanced by the drug and, moreover, that the dose–response curve interacted with strain in such a way that the TMB group had a lower optimum dose (0.50 mg/kg) than the maze dulls (0.75 mg/kg), at which the latter outperformed the brights so that the usual strain difference was in fact reversed. The authors interpret this effect as a stimulatory one, beneficially affecting a consolidation process directly, but, as we shall see, the more recent view is that the cholinergic system has a generally depressive behavioral effect in reducing activity and avoidance learning. It may be this aspect that accounts for the effects found, in that reduced activity diminished behaviors liable to interfere with consolidation processes. In a further contribution from this group, Burt (1962) studied a drug response different from those we have previously been considering—the seizure threshold to daily increasing doses of picrotoxin until fatal levels were reached. While the TMD strain was more resistant to athetotic movements and convulsions than the TMB, the TMD rats had a lower dose threshold for fatal seizures.

Powell *et al.* (1967) used the Tryon strains to test the effect of amobarbital on their escape–avoidance conditioning, having first established that the TMBs showed greater emotional reactivity than the TMDs in open-field measures (greater defecation and less ambulation), though these measures were derived from a single day's testing, which lessens their validity. Both of the dosages used (20 and 40 mg/kg) depressed the performance of the maze-dull rats when injected 20 min prior to testing on each of the five days on which 20 trials were given, but only the larger dose had the same effect on the maze-bright rats. The 20-mg/kg dose augmented their performance to such an extent that a significant dose–strain interaction was detected. The authors' explanation of the strain difference in terms of emotionality variables is out of keeping with the usual finding in that more emotional rats tend to do *less* well in avoidance response acquisition (Broadhurst, 1975).

In contrast to the considerable study of alcohol preference in other selected strains, as we shall see, the Tryon strains have been little used in this connection. Indeed, only one published study (Russell and Stern, 1973) has come to hand in which they were examined alongside two other strains of unstated provenance for their acceptance of ethanol solution in daily increasing concentrations in preference to water. The TMB group showed a higher final concentration than the TMD group, together with a contrast in the significant sex differences found, females being higher in the former and lower in the latter. If replicable, these differences may prove very useful in further analyses of their genetic bases. Fortunately, data are now available which bear on this point. Drewek and Broadhurst (1978) included the TMB and TMD strains in a survey of rat strains in a carefully designed experiment on alcohol preference, using a range of six concentrations presented sequentially over a period of six weeks—one per week—using the three-bottle two-choice technique of Myers and Holman (1966). This method insures that position habit artifacts do not disturb recorded preferences, since the inclusion of a dry nozzle, the relative position of which was varied daily, forces the subject to sample the two other tubes containing water or the alcohol to determine its choice. Controls for changes in fluid consumption over time and for spillage and evaporation were also included. The six concentrations used were 2%, 4%, 6%, 8%, 10%, and 12% (wt./vol.), thus spanning the range from near threshold for taste to aversion levels. Drewek and Broadhurst showed that for measures of preference—percentage of daily fluid intake represented by the alcohol solution—the results, especially at the higher concentrations, supported the findings of Russell and Stern (1973) that the maze-bright rats showed a markedly higher preference than the dulls (TMD), and the females of that strain were, in turn, more preferring than the males. Another measure employed, that of the daily alcohol intake, showed similar results for the TMBs, with the TMD group's data yielding an even more marked optimum concentration effect on this measure than they did for the other. This was seen in an increase in intake up to a concentration of 6% (wt./vol.) followed by a decrease at the higher values (10% and 12%). A third measure taken, that of alcohol calorie contribution, made possible by comparisons with dry food intake, gave a congruent picture. Sleep time in response to a 3-g/kg intraperitoneal injection of 30% (wt./vol.) alcohol showed no difference between the two strains.

The use of subjects from the Tryon selection experiment—one of the most practical legacies from a distinguished period in the history of American psychology—has not been especially productive in the light in which we have chosen to consider it here. Despite the inherent possibility that this valuable biological material offers for genetic analysis of psychopharmacological phenotypes—as well as many others, of course—little advantage has been taken of their potentialities in this connection. The analysis we have been able to present was based on data cobbled together from different experiments and its obvious limitations reflect this fact. One sometimes has the impression that the Tryon strains were used merely because they were available and less because of their intrinsic interest. Moreover, the line of research—that of experimentally modifying neural processes by pharmacological means in order to study the basis of memory—for which they were largely used has perhaps passed its peak of interest in view of the difficulty of establishing the neurobiological bases of the effects observed (McGaugh, 1973). But maybe these judgments are a little harsh, especially when it is borne in mind that in the early 1960s behavioral genetics, or psychogenetics as it is sometimes called, had hardly come to establish itself as a recognized specialization within psychology in the United States, so the possibilities of its cross-fertilization with another, though somewhat longer established specialization, psychopharmacology, could not have been expected to be recognized.

We now turn our attention to a second selection experiment that has been used in psychopharmacology. Bignami and Bovet (1965; Bignami, 1965) describe the foundation of the Roman strains of rats, which now comprise the *R*oman *h*igh-*a*voidance strain (RHA), the *l*ow-*a*voidance strain (RLA), and a control strain, the RCA, which is maintained as an unselected control line deriving from the same general Wistar stock. They were founded in Rome, where the first five generations were selected for speed of acquisition of two-way escape–avoidance conditioning, using shock as the unconditioned stimulus and light as the conditioned stimulus. After the S_5 generation, the experiment was continued at Birmingham (Broadhurst and Bignami, 1965), where a buzzer replaced light as the conditioned stimulus. Progress of selection to the S_{13} generation has been documented by Fleming and Broadhurst (1975); good separation had been achieved between the strains.

A body of psychopharmacological work has employed these strains, as may be seen from the summary in Table VI. In early studies at their laboratory of origin, Bignami *et al.* (1965) showed that the low-avoidance strain (RLA) responded with improved performance to 0.5 mg/kg of amphetamine sulfate given subcutaneously 30 min before test sessions of avoidance conditioning. This effect was confirmed by Coyle *et al.* (1973), the same size dose of *d*-amphetamine being given intraperitoneally one hour before testing in a shuttle box comparable with that used in selection, resulting in a distinct improvement in performance as compared with saline controls from the same strain. Since only one strain was employed to examine the drug response in both of these studies, the extent to which this effect is strain dependent only became clear in subsequent work.

Thus, Satinder (1971) showed that *d*-amphetamine, far from enhancing avoidance performance in the high-avoidance (RHA) strain, either had little effect at the lower dosages given (1.0 and 2.0 mg/kg i.p. 30 min before the commencement of a block of ten trials) or caused a marked decline in performance at the higher doses (3.0 and 4.0 mg/kg). The latter, not surprisingly, had similar effects on the RLA, but the lower dosages, especially 1.0 mg/kg, improved mean performance. Other measures derived from the same test, such as avoidance and escape response latencies, showed no comparable drug–strain interaction, though intertrial crossings, a measure of spontaneous activity in this situation, did. Here it was the RHA group that showed a marked increase in response to the two lower dosages, which strengthens the confidence that can be placed in the finding relating to the absence of improvement in learning in this strain—since it suggests that the positive finding for the other (RLA) strain is not primarily an artifact of increased activity. This reassurance is doubly welcome in view of the absence in this report of details of the analyses of variance on which such conclusions could otherwise be based. The question was further examined (Satinder, 1972*b*) in a study which may have employed some of the data from the male subjects of the previous report, but which extended the training period to include sessions during which intertrial crossings were punished by shock. The same doses of amphetamine as before were augmented by a lower one, 0.5 mg/kg, making five in all. As might be expected, the macroenvironmental variation represented by the punishment for intertrial crossing itself interacted with the strain-dependent drug effect found before, in that the increase in avoidance responding occasioned by the lower doses and limited to the RLA strain was suppressed.

In further work on amphetamine, Satinder and Petryshyn (1974) used a one-way jump-up avoidance conditioning procedure in which the Roman strains differed, though somewhat less than with respect to the two-way running procedure for which they are selectively bred. But the response to *d*-amphetamine sulfate in four dose levels (0.5, 1.0, 2.0, and 4.0 mg/kg) plus a placebo was broadly the same as for two-way responding. In six separate experiments the performance of the RHAs was either depressed, especially at the higher doses, or did not improve, whereas the RLA rats generally showed some positive response. In some cases this difference is reflected in the absence of statistical significance between the strains, which had previously existed during the training period before the drug was given. Also, strain–drug-dosage interactions from the appropriate ANOVA are sometimes reported as significant. In another experiment, Satinder (1977*b*) compared the strains in yet a further conditioning procedure in which rats were allowed freedom of choice as to the direction they ran in response to the same conditioned and unconditioned stimuli as in the standard two-way avoidance conditioning previously used, and in a one-way arrangement requiring the same running response. The data showed that this latter arrangement was even easier to learn in all strains than the other two men-

TABLE VI

Pharmacology and Psychogenetic Selection: The Roman Rat Strains

Reference	Treatment	Measure	Outcome	Remarks
Bignami et al. (1965)	Amphetamine 30 min before	Escape-avoidance conditioning	Improved	RLA only
Coyle et al. (1973)	Amphetamine 1 hr before	Shuttle box	Improved	RLA only
		Catecholamine levels	Enzymatic activity lower in RLA adrenals	
Satinder (1971)	Amphetamine 30 min before	Escape-avoidance conditioning	Low doses improved RLA, high gave drug–strain interaction	
		Intertrial activity	Drug–strain interaction	
Satinder (1972b)	Amphetamine 30 min before	Intertrial activity, punished	RLA increase with low dose suppressed	
Satinder and Petryshyn (1974)	Amphetamine	One-way avoidance	Similar to two-way	
Buxton (1974), Brimblecome et al. (1975)	Amphetamine 30 min before	Spontaneous activity	RLA greater response	
Satinder (1977b)	Amphetamine	One-, two-, and either-way avoidance conditioning	RLA improved more. No reciprocal difference in drug effects	F_1 included
Buxton (1974)	Physostigmine immediately before	Activity	Larger doses interact with strain	
	Pyridostigmine	Activity	No effect	
	NEPB	Activity	Drug–strain interaction RLA more affected	
	NEPB-MeI	Activity	No effect	
	Physostigmine	Escape-avoidance conditioning	Larger doses interact with strain	"Floor" effect?
	Pyridostigmine + NEPB	Escape-avoidance conditioning	n.s. effect; RLA improved	"Ceiling" effect?
	NEPB-MeI	Escape-avoidance conditioning	Responding generally depressed	
	NEPB + Amphetamine	Escape-avoidance conditioning	Enhanced avoidance in RLA	Small doses ineffective separately
	Amphetamine 15 min	Escape-avoidance	Stimulated all three strains	

Reference	Treatment	Measure	Result	Comments
Buxton et al. (1976)		Brain acetylcholine and acetylcholinesterase assay	No strain difference in acetylcholinesterase; RLA acetylcholine > Wistar > RHA	
Satinder (1971)	Caffeine 30 min before	Escape-avoidance conditioning	Only RHA intertrial activity increased significantly	
Brewster (1969)	Alcohol preference	Four different concentrations	Only 7.9% (wt./vol.) solution differentiates	Confirmed by Satinder (1972a)
Satinder (1975)	Alcohol preference	Effect with age	Only RHA increased	
Drewek and Broadhurst (1978)	Alcohol preference	Six different concentrations	RHA prefer, RCA, RLA aversive	
Gregory (1967)	Alcohol injection	Sleep time	n.s. difference	
Satinder (1977a)	Methylpentynol	Rearing	n.s. effect	
	Morphine	Preference over quinine after habituation	RHA and RLA > RCA	RLAs now showing preference
Satinder (personal communication, 1974)	Morphine	Preference after 21-day abstinence	n.s. difference	
Satinder (1976)	Morphine 1–96 hr before	Escape-avoidance conditioning	RHA > RCA > RLA	
Garg (1968, 1969c)	Nicotine 15 min before	Rearing, frequency	RHA increased	High dose!
Garg (1968, 1969c)	Nicotine 15 min before	Rearing, duration	n.s. effect	High dose!
Garg (1969, 1969c), Garg and Holland (1969)	Nicotine 2 min after	Hebb–Williams maze, errors	Report unclear	High dose!
Bovet-Nitti (1966)	Nicotine 15 min before	Visual discrimination	Some improvement	Females only
Keenan and Johnson (1972)	Nicotine 20 min before	Rearing	Significantly reduced at first	RCA only
Bignami et al. (1965)	Nicotine 10 min before	Escape-avoidance conditioning	Significantly improved	RLA only
Garg (1969a)	Nicotine 2 min after	Escape-avoidance conditioning	n.s. effects	Single daily trials!
Fleming and Broadhurst (1975)	Nicotine 0–30 min before	Escape-avoidance conditioning	n.s. effects, except on activity	Included RCA
	Nicotine before	Operant conditioning	Increased	
Bättig et al. (1976)	Nicotine 35 min before	Locomotor activity in maze	Increased	Drug–strain interaction?
Driscoll (1976)	Nicotine 30 min before	Escape-avoidance latency	Facilitated extinction	RHA only
	Mecamylamine 30 min before	Escape-avoidance latency	Facilitated extinction	RHA only

tioned, which were confirmed as being descending in order of difficulty. Using almost the same range of doses of amphetamine as before, except that the 0.5 mg/kg level was omitted, he showed that, once again, the low-avoidance RLA strain benefited more from amphetamine than did the other two strains—the highs and the controls. This effect is enhanced in both one-way and the new either-way situations, so much so that the avoidance scores of the low strain under the drug dosages used are virtually indistinguishable from those of the high strain in the latter. The fact that this is also true under the placebo condition as well suggested a longer-term action of the drug than had previously been suspected, since the doses were given in balanced order, but this explanation can be ruled out because rats receiving the placebo before any amphetamine at all did not differ from those that did. A strain-limited reminiscence effect from training to testing remains a possibility that would, of course, confound the drug response detected. An extension of this work to the jump-up one-way procedure previously used showed a reversal of the standing of the high- and low-avoidance strains with respect to avoidance scores during training, though they became similar under amphetamine, which casts some doubt on Satinder and Petryshyn's (1974) findings. Of more interest in the present context is a report on a small group of 32 first-filial (F_1) crosses between them. These crosses were made reciprocally and the resultant offspring given the same one- and two-way, though not the either-way, conditioning procedures and drug treatment as described above. The resulting data are useful, primarily for the clear demonstration of the absence of reciprocal differences in drug effects on avoidance responses that they present. There was some suggestion of reciprocal differences in another score, escape latency, but these results were confined to the two-way avoidance task, and do not markedly detract from the overall impression of the absence of important prenatal maternal effects (see Section 9.1) in these drug–strain interactions. The phenotypic scores of the two F_1 groups thus generated showed essentially similar dose–response relationships to those of the two parental strains, though there was some suggestion, especially in the two-way task, that they resembled the low-avoidance strain more than the high-avoidance strain. This indication of potence (see Chapter 6) for low avoidance does not, of course, allow inferences about the genetic dominance of controlling genes.

It seems clear that the differential strain-limited response to amphetamine in the Roman strains can be regarded as reasonably well established, especially since Buxton (1974; Buxton *et al.*, 1976; Brimble-combe *et al.*, 1975) reported that the RLA strain shows a greater response than the RHA to a single dose of *d*-amphetamine, small (0.1 mg/kg) compared with those Satinder and his colleague used, and that the time course of the response suggested a maximal differentiation between the strains between 30 and 40 min after administration, precisely the time interval during which performance was being measured in Satinder's work. That the response being measured, however, was not conditioned responding but an increase in spontaneous activity suggests that the problem of the causal relationship between the two behaviors is not yet fully resolved. Following this with an interesting synergistic experiment, Buxton combined the administration of *d*-amphetamine, in a subcutaneous dose (0.075 mg/kg), which he had previously shown did not affect activity, with a similarly silent intraperitoneal dose of *N*-ethyl-3-piperidyl benzilate (NEPB) (0.75 mg/kg), an atropine-like (i.e., antimuscarinic) anticholinergic, which together gave significantly higher activity levels 70 and 80 min postinjection than those found among rats given either drug separately, or a saline control. But the subjects for this demonstration of the combinatorial effects of the two drugs were not the Roman strains, but a random-bred Wistar-derived strain used, in this and Buxton's subsequent work, as a substitute for the RCA or unselected Roman strain more usually employed, for example, by Fleming and Broadhurst (1975), as a control or reference strain in conjunction with the RHA and RLA. These two strains were, however, included in an impressive series of investigations of the effects on activity of other compounds, chosen for the light that their action might throw on, first, cholinergic systems and, second, the balance between them in the Roman strains. These are, in relation to the first, the anticholinesterases, physostigmine salicylate and pyridostigmine hydrobromide (the latter being a drug whose action, unlike that of physostigmine, is believed to be more of an antagonist of acetylcholinesterase at peripheral rather than central sites). Two drugs that fulfill the second role act against acetylcholine itself (rather than against its catabolic or hydrolytic enzyme), again, in one case, centrally as well as peripherally—NEPB (see above), and its quaternary congener *N*-ethyl-3-piperidyl-benzilate methiodide (NEPB-MeI), which would be expected to act only peripherally against acetylcholinesterase since it penetrates the blood–brain barrier only poorly. This approach combined with regional and other brain assays of acetylcholine and acetylcholinesterase in the three rat strains constitutes a powerful pharmacogenetic tool of a more sophisticated kind than the earlier (but not dissimilar) attempts to devise a "four-drug paradigm" to be discussed later.

The impact of this patterning of agents was assessed by means of the activity measure already referred to as well as by two-way escape–avoidance conditioning of a kind with that used in the selection of the Roman strains. As regards activity, it was found that, compared with control (saline) injected rats, the lower doses of physostigmine (0.125 mg/kg) injected immediately before recording began produced little in the way of significant effects, whereas the larger dose (0.25 mg/kg) showed an interaction with strain. The RHA showed a relatively profound depression, whereas the RLA were less affected and the Wistar control strain showed not only a very short-lived diminution in activity, but subsequently some measure of hyperactivity. Pyridostigmine (0.125 mg/kg), on the other hand, had no effects reaching significance by the methods of analysis used throughout this work, which were not perhaps the most efficient in that comparisons were made within strains and never between strains as well, so that the significance of interaction effects was not formally assessed. Also, the analysis did not extend to taking account of the trend in the data with the passage of time. The antiacetylcholine drug, NEPB, yielded a similar drug–strain interaction in that the degree of hyperactivity induced in all the strains by the two doses used (2.0 and 1.0 mg/kg) varied as between the strains and also differed in detail. The RLA strain was maximally affected, especially by the lower dose, and the RHA strain less so, with the Wistar control showing only a transitory effect. Again the putatively peripherally acting compound, NEPB-MeI, had no significant effects in the single dosage used (1.0 mg/kg).

The application of this methodology to avoidance conditioning also yielded data full of interest (Buxton, 1974). Physostigmine in the larger two of the three doses (0.125, 0.06, and 0.03 mg/kg) given 15 min before the first four of five daily sessions, each comprised of 50 trials, had pronounced depressive effects as measured by an increase in the number of failures to make even escape responses to shock in the shuttle box, and in decreasing the number of successful avoidance responses. In each case the comparison was to saline controls. That the latter effect was less pronounced in the normally low-avoidance strain than in the RHA and Wistar strains is probably the result of their undrugged low performance, that is, a "floor effect" may be masquerading as a drug–strain interaction. Peripheral action again could be discounted by the absence of significant effects of pyridostigmine in a single dose of 0.125 mg/kg. These findings, together with those relating to activity measures discussed above, led Buxton to expect that treatment with the antiacetylcholine compound, NEPB, would lead to stimulatory effects on avoidance learning. Such indeed was the case, the effects of the single dose used (1.0 mg/kg) being especially dramatic in the RLA strain in that not only was escape behavior (unconditioned responding to the shock) enhanced, but levels of avoidance responding were observed to be significantly greater than the zero level returned by the saline controls. Once again it is difficult to assess the extent of the drug–strain interaction in the absence of analysis appropriate for that purpose, and again there may be an artifactual complication—in this case a "ceiling effect" for the high-avoidance strain whose performance is such that little improvement in it is possible, at least in the later sessions—but the impression may be gained that, if present, the interaction is not marked. The effects of NEPB-MeI (dose 1.0 mg/kg) were also assessed with the somewhat anomalous outcome that responding was generally depressed, a finding that was attributed to an increase in skin resistance and hence to a decrease in the aversive power of the shock used in avoidance conditioning. This interpretation was confirmed in experimentation that showed a significant increase in the flinch threshold to shock in rats of all three strains when given NEPB-MeI, but not its tertiary counterpart, NEPB. No strain differences or interactions were noted. These findings for the two antiacetylcholine agents were mirrored in measures of extinction of avoidance responding, using only RHA and Wistar strains. The former showed a delayed decline with unreinforced trials under NEPB, which reached significant proportions on the last three days of six daily sessions of 20 trials each. NEPB-MeI had minor nonsignificant depressive effects on performance.

The combinatory effect of NEPB and amphetamine was also investigated, using the same two dosages noted above, in relation to their effects on activity, which were equally inactive as regards avoidance conditioning. Buxton showed that together they had an enhancing effect on the acquisition of avoidance behavior, and that this effect was probably strain-dependent in that the RHA animals were relatively unaffected in contrast to the Wistar and low-avoidance strains, which showed significant increases in the efficiency of learning in several of the sessions. Finally, the effect of amphetamine alone (0.1 mg/kg injected subcutaneously 15 min before the start of four out of five daily sessions) was shown to be stimulatory in all three strains, the effect being especially marked, and, of course, fully significant in the first three sessions of the RHA strain—in contrast to Satinder's negative finding (1971) discussed earlier—and expressing itself among rats of the RLA strain as an increase in the number of successful escape responses.

These findings are supported by extensive analyses of the levels of brain acetylcholine and acetylcholinesterase activity in the three strains, both before and, in the first case, after administration of the drugs used in the behavioral work. They may be summarized by noting that no important differences were detected with respect to acetylcholinesterase, but that acetylcholine concentration was shown to be strain-dependent: The low-avoidance strain had significantly higher whole-brain values than the high-avoidance group, with the Wistar strain being intermediate. Regional assays gave congruent results, with the hypothalamus having the highest concentrations, followed by the midbrain region, with medulla and cortex being intermediate, and cerebellum lowest. The RLA strain exceeded the RHA strain significantly for each area except in the case of the midbrain. The changes occasioned in these values by the drugs injected 30 min before sacrificing animals had effects on brain acetylcholine in directions to be anticipated from the behavioral observations, with physostigmine causing increases in all three strains and NEPB decreases, and their analogs, as well as amphetamine, giving no significant differences. Some regional variations in concentration, taken together with the strain differences referred to above, led Buxton to suggest that, first, the ratio of acetylcholine to its metabolic enzyme acetylcholinesterase may be larger in the RLA rats than in the RHAs, from which it follows that, second, the two may not be genetically linked. This latter point can, of course, only be satisfactorily resolved by methods involving the crossbreeding of filial generations in which the phenotypic response to drugs is also examined, as in, for example, the work of Anisman, to be considered later (see Sections 5.2 and 6).

The absence of biochemical effects of *d*-amphetamine on the cholinergic systems investigated by Buxton emphasizes the known adrenergic systemic action of this drug. This conclusion was reinforced by the neurochemical investigations of Coyle *et al.* (1973) into the catecholamine levels in the RHA and RLA strains, using another Wistar-derived strain, this time the Sprague–Dawley, as a third control strain. The activity of various catecholamine synthesizing enzymes was determined to be significantly lower in the adrenal glands of the RLAs, congruent with their lower response to stress as observed in their poor avoidance performance and low activity. On the other hand, this strain does not differ from the RHA strain with respect to norepinephrine turnover in the brain, and the authors conclude that ". . . the concurrence between the biochemical and behavioral studies do [sic] not support the hypothesis of a generalized disturbance of the central catecholaminergic neurons in the RLAs" (Coyle *et al.* 1973, p. 33).

Resuming the more directly psychopharmacological approach, it may be noted that caffeine has also been studied for its effects on two-way conditioning in these strains by Satinder (1971), using the same paradigms as for *d*-amphetamine with no significant effects on performance and no suggestion of differential response between the high and low rats except for intertrial activity, which increased significantly among the RHA animals.

Nicotine is a drug that has been much studied in the context of the Roman strains selection. Bignami *et al.* (1965) investigated its effect in a single dose level of 0.2 mg/kg [along with those of delysid (0.1), benactyzine chlorhydrate (5.0), *n*-ethyl-3-piperidyl cyclopentenylphenyl glycolate or Ditran (5.0)] and found significant stimulation on the performance of the RLA strain, no comparison being possible with the RHA strain which was not tested in the same experiment. Bovet-Nitti (1966), using females of the two strains, showed that in response to a subcutaneous injection of 0.2 mg/kg of nicotine sulfate 15 min before a visual discrimination task they both improved performance but in one only of three experiments. The technique used is described more fully later in connection with work with mice (see Section 7.1). Garg has reported extensively on experiments using nicotine on these strains, often using a single, very high dose (0.8 mg/kg), of nicotine tartrate injected, for example, 15 min prior to a rearing test, in which the animals' vertical movements were automatically recorded by means of a proximity meter sensing changes in electrical capacitance in a cylindrical chamber. She showed that only the RHA strain increased their frequency of rearing, but there was no similar drug–strain interaction with respect to the duration of the rearing, which suggests that the high-avoidance strain merely increased their up and down activity (Garg, 1968, 1969c). Keenan and Johnson (1972) demonstrated the development of tolerance in the effects of daily nicotine (0.5 mg/kg) on rearing but in the control (RCA) strain only. Battig *et al.* (1976) used females only of both the selected strains and examined their locomotor activity in a complex maze pattern in response to 0.2 mg/kg of nicotine tartrate injected subcutaneous-ly 35 min before the 6 min exposure to one of the six different maze patterns used. In the absence of the report of the application of ANOVA techniques, it is not possible to be certain if drug–strain interactions were detected. The results reported suggest a rather general proportionate increase in activity measures of various kinds, though the authors claim some degree of greater response among the RHA group, especially when tested at night—the diur-nal rat's waking period—as compared with daytime, a valuable feature of this investigation.

Consolidation hypotheses were also investigated by means of im-mediate posttrial injections of 0.8 mg/kg of nicotine in two rather different situations. In the Hebb–Williams maze (Garg, 1969a; Garg and Holland, 1969) the subjects were treated 2 min after daily trials 6 through 15, run for a food reward. Presentation of the results makes it difficult to assess the details of the significant drug–strain interaction appearing in the ANOVA. A study of avoidance conditioning, begun 14 days after the maze learning had ended (Garg, 1969a), extended over 15 days, with 5 days of 5 min per day of preliminary exploration of the shuttle box followed by 10 single daily trials under the same regimen of 2-min posttrial nicotine or placebo injec-tions. This highly unusual approach to escape-avoidance conditioning perhaps guaranteed the absence of any significant differences whatsoever in either avoidance or latency scores—even between the Roman strains selected for their response to this situation. It is just possible that the previous experience of the maze may have contributed to this anomalous result, which may be contrasted with Satinder's and Petryshyn's demonstra-tion (1974) of the generalizability of the RHA and RLA strains' differential status to one-way as opposed to two-way avoidance.

And there the matter of the increase in RLA scores under nicotine shown by Bignami *et al.* (1965) rested until Fleming and Broadhurst (1975) reported a large-scale study using both strains and the RCA or unselected control strain, which were injected subcutaneously with a placebo or one of a series of five doses ranging from 0.05 to 0.8 mg/kg at three time intervals (0, 15, or 30 min) before a single session of 30 trials of two-way avoidance conditioning. While the usual strain differences were detected, no effect of dose level or delay interval could be demonstrated on avoidance acquisition, though latencies and activity scores showed some interactions with sex and with strain. The score for presessional activity showed that the RLA group did not display the increase at the lower dose levels seen in both the other strains, before all three fell off at the highest dose levels. The sensitivity of both RHA and RLA rats to the effects of a single dose of 0.2 mg/kg on operant behavior was demonstrated without any marked drug–strain interaction. Clearly, any confirmation of the effect of nicotine on avoidance behavior in the RLA strain in the way that has been demonstrated for amphetamine is still awaited. Driscoll's demonstration (1976) that doses of 0.1 and 0.2 mg/kg shorten avoidance latencies does not assist, since it was confined to RHA rats and dealt with latencies during avoidance extinction procedures. Interestingly enough, however, it did show that mecamylamine, often used as a central antagonist of nicotine, can, at least in the smaller of the two doses used (0.25 and 0.5 mg/kg), have a facilitating effect on these rats' extinction latencies, comparable with that of nicotine.

The effect of an anxiolytic, methylpentynol carbamate, on the Roman strains was investigated by Gregory (1967). He found that while the experience of shock between two trials in the rearing apparatus significantly depressed scores on the second trial, neither the effect of the drug nor the strain was evident. In another investigation (Gregory, 1968a) involving the measure of rearing, there was no possibility of the detection of drug–strain interaction since only the high-avoidance strain (RHA) was studied. Prenylamine and reserpine in the highest doses used (4.0 and 40.0 mg/kg, respectively) significantly suppressed both activity as well as the acquisition of escape–avoidance conditioning. Though the essential comparison with the RLA rats was lacking, it was argued that these findings supported the notion that the difference between these selected strains was partly based on differences in their activity.

Preference phenotypes have also been investigated. Brewster (1969) studied the preference of the three Roman strains (RHA, RLA, and RCA) for four different concentrations of ethanol solutions, but found that only the highest used, 7.9% (wt./vol.) unequivocally differentiated them either with respect to percentage preference or to intake—two of the measures also used by Drewek and Broadhurst (1978) in their investigations using the

Tryon strains, as discussed earlier. Brewster found that the high-avoidance strain was significantly higher than either the RLA or the controls on both measures. Satinder (1972*a*) broadly confirmed these findings in three experiments using various preference concentrations and various environmental manipulations, including a sustained period (three weeks) of forced consumption followed by alcohol deprivation lasting one week. The RHA rats not only showed a higher mean intake throughout, but significantly increased their intake after the forced abstinence, which neither of the other strains did. Response to food deprivation as measured by increased preference for a 7.9% ethanol solution did not differentiate the strains especially clearly, except that the RCA group showed less response than the other two, and the RHA group showed a tendency toward greater overall consumption. In further work along the same lines, Satinder (1975) used only the high and low strains in an experiment designed to study the effect of age on preference, finding that only the former, the RHA, increased with age. In a second experiment, which included the RCA controls, the strains were studied over an extended period (more than 20 weeks), during which subjects were allowed either water or a 7.9% (wt./vol.) solution only, and preference was measured biweekly except at the end. Weight and open-field test data were also collected. Strain differences were not especially prominent, though the previously observed tendency of the RHA strain toward greater alcohol consumption was sustained.

Once again, Drewek and Broadhurst (1978) provide data that bear on the marked preference for alcohol displayed by the RHA rats. Using the range of concentrations and the three-bottle two-choice technique described earlier, they were able to confirm that this is a high-preferring strain, with preference ratios approaching 80% for both males and females at the 4% (wt./vol.) concentration, after which there is a definite decline so that by the time the highest concentration (12% wt./vol.) was reached, less than 50% of the rats' daily fluid intake was coming from the alcohol solution. Thus they display an optimal preference, probably based on a relatively acute sensitivity to the drug. Other measures (alcohol intake and calorie contribution) yield data that support this view. The RLA and RCA strains, on the other hand, are confirmed as relatively aversive to alcohol. Only at the lower concentrations (2% and 4% wt./vol.) does the preference measure show any degree of acceptance, after which a sustained decline with increasing concentration is seen. The other two measures Drewek and Broadhurst used show relative stability or slight increases with concentration. As with the Tryon strains, no differences in sleep time in response to injected alcohol were found.

Preference methods have been extended to the study of another phenotype, self-administration of morphine (Satinder, 1977*a*) after a regimen not unlike that used for establishing the morphine-directed behavior previously encountered in Nichols' selection experiment (see Chapter 3), except that morphine was not injected directly, but consumption was forced by offering morphine in increasingly strong concentrations with, at first, decreasing sucrose concentrations (used in the early stages to mask its bitter taste). Two-day preference tests were given immediately after each level of increasing morphine concentration, except for the last (1.2 mg/ml), before which two days abstinence was imposed. The whole procedure occupied 50 days. The RHA strain showed higher consumption of morphine throughout, as compared with the other two strains, and clear evidence of a gradual increase in proportional preference during the course of the increasing progression of doses, together with an increase in preference for the highest concentration after the two-day withdrawal that preceded this test. These data contrast with the RLA strain's behavior which, while showing some degree of increasing preference, actually decreased its preference after the withdrawal period, and the RCA strain, which showed no increase in preference at all. In a further experiment (Satinder, personal communication, 1974), the same subjects were subjected to a second enforced abstinence, this time lasting 21 days, after which two further two-day preference tests were given before and after a forced consumption period of morphine in the highest concentration. Here no strain differences were found, and levels of consumption were generally lower, which was interpreted as indicating no tendency to respond to withdrawal by enhanced intake.

In addition, Satinder used the Roman strains in a second experiment (Satinder, 1977*a*) in which a control for taste aversion was introduced. Quinine in a concentration of 0.25 mg/ml was shown to be equally aversive when compared with water in a two-bottle preference test, as was 0.5 mg/ml of morphine sulfate. These single doses were used throughout a long (58 day) period of intermittent exposure to two drug groups, during which seven cycles of five days of forced drinking and two days of preference testing preceded a final cycle in which a two-day period of both food and water deprivation was interposed before the final preference testing. Comparisons were made between these groups and a further control group in which the rats were given water throughout, except, of course, during preference tests for morphine. The results confirmed the significantly greater susceptibility of the RHA strain to morphine as shown by the increasing preference seen in the first experiment, but not shared and even exceeded by the RLA group. The control strain (RCA), by contrast, was unequivocally confirmed as being a low-preference strain. Among all three selected strains, the control groups given quinine or water throughout showed uniformly lower morphine preference.

Satinder (1976) has also investigated the effects of morphine as such on avoidance responses, using an increasing (doubling) dose twice daily for five days, so that the initial 14 mg/kg of morphine sulfate (i.p.) reached 224 mg/kg on the morning of the fifth day. Testing for two-way escape–avoidance conditioning then followed at four intervals ranging from 1 to 96 hr, separate groups of rats being used for each determination of acquisition of the response in a single session of 30 trials. Placebo (saline injected) and noninjected controls were also used, but the report does not make clear when they were tested. However, care was taken to equate the shock level in the shuttle apparatus over the various groups, though this procedure could have resulted in differential preshock exposure that may have affected later learning. The avoidance data are very orderly (RHA > RCA > RLA) for the control group, though not for the placebo group, in which the RHA and RCA share the same relatively high values. The effect of morphine varied with time, showing a clear depression of all group scores after the first, 1-hr post-final-injection, test. At this time, the low-avoidance group (RLA) exceeded both the RHA and the RCA, though intertrial crossing did not differ significantly, which led Satinder to conclude that differences in activity due to morphine withdrawal were unlikely to have influenced the results. But when one bears in mind that the three strains were represented by four subjects only from each strain, perhaps a little more emphasis should be placed on these fluctuations than upon the paradoxical facilitation of the RLA scores in the injection–control group noted above. Somewhat subjective appraisal of various indices of the systemic effect of morphine, as well as fatalities due to it, are noted as showing some interactions with strain.

In reviewing the work on pharmacological phenotypes as studied in the Roman selection strains (Table VI), we find no examples of data amenable to the biometrical analyses of the kind available for the Tryon strains (Table V). On the other hand, it is probably true to say that there is a wider range and greater volume of data, which may well provide a more secure base for such analyses when they come to be attempted. In particular, Buxton's and Satinder's work demonstrating the facilitatory effect of amphetamine on the low-avoidance RLA strain, and the latter's work on the higher preference of the high-avoidance RHA strain for drugs of dependence are of considerable interest and will, if further confirmed, give that essential foundation of reliable interstrain differences without which crossbreeding studies, designed to explore the genetic architecture of the phenotype in question, cannot proceed.

A third selection experiment has also been of some prominence in studying pharmacological phenotypes in the rat. This is the selective breeding for extremes of emotional elimination (defecation) in the open-field test of Hall (1934), which resulted in the establishment in 1954 of the Maudsley strains, known as the MR or *M*audsley *r*eactive and the MNR or *M*audsley *n*onreactive. The designation now adopted refers solely to the responsivity to the stimulation offered the rat by the mild stress of noise, light, and space of the open-field arena. The development of these strains and their use in other centers is chronicled by Broadhurst (1958, 1960, 1962, 1975; Eysenck and Broadhurst, 1964). The strains are characterized by striking and consistent differences in the defecation measure for which they were selected, the MR being higher and the MNR lower, and in the inversely correlated response—not selected for—of ambulation in the open field, the MNR rats being the higher in this respect. Evidence reviewed in the references above (especially Broadhurst, 1975) suggests a valid differentiation between the strains in a general emotionality or emotional reactivity, though this view is further discussed in Archer's critique (1975) and the reply thereto (Broadhurst, 1976).

The following survey of psychopharmacological studies on these strains, which is summarized in Table VII, will to some extent recapitulate that presented above for the Roman strains since in some investigations both sets of selectively bred strains served as subjects. Experimental details will not be repeated in such cases and the reader should refer back to the description given in the text at the first citation.

The "four-drug paradigm" was used in several investigations with these strains and stems from the period when Eysenck's "drug postulate" (1957, p. 229) was especially in vogue. It is important to note that the postulate was a corollary of his "typological postulate," which was concerned not with animal behavior but with the basic processes underlying personality dimensions in humans, and related primarily to individual differences in introversion–extraversion. No one concerned with the comparative aspects sought to identify the differences exemplified by the two Maudsley strains of rats as constituting an animal analog of introversion–extraversion in humans; indeed, such claims as were made—and they were relatively muted (Broadhurst and Eysenck, 1965)—suggested rather that "emotionality" in rats was more akin to the autonomic instability thought to be a substrate of emotional lability of human neuroticism, a dimension probably orthogonal to introversion–extraversion. Be that as it may, there was nevertheless an enthusiasm for using drugs as tools to quarry the control of behavior, the approach adopted was logically sound and, of its time, technically advanced, if simplistic in its assumptions. It was perhaps most clearly expressed by Singh (1961) in a paper that does not altogether merit the oblivion that has overtaken its publication in a journal not widely consulted in the West. All the more reason, therefore, to quote from it:

Pharmacologically, there are drugs which are classified into two categories: drugs mainly affecting the higher central nervous system, and known as central stimulants and depressants, and drugs mainly affecting the autonomic nervous system, and known as autonomic stimulants and depressants. For the study of the underlying mechanism of [behavior], it seems important to know which of the two types of drugs, central or autonomic, has greater effect. There is little available evidence bearing on this problem. It seems, therefore, that the use of both stimulant and depressant drugs which, broadly speaking, are known for their action at either the central or autonomic level might be helpful for this purpose. This implies a fourfold classification of drugs of the type shown in Table 1. It must be stressed that this classification of drugs is arbitrary, because the site of action of a drug is frequently not well established. It is only adopted here to provide an approximation to a rational basis for selection of the drugs actually used. (p. 1)

Singh's table, to which I have added in parentheses the names of other drugs substituted in this paradigm at other times for various experiments by other workers in the Maudsley group or associated with it, is presented as Table VIII.

Occasionally, only half the paradigm was used, usually according to "level" (central or autonomic) as is exemplified in some of the earliest work using the selected Maudsley strains as subjects. Thus Sinha *et al.* (1958) sought to test the prediction that the Maudsley emotionally reactive (MR) rats would show less alternation in a maze than the MNR or nonreactives, and that this behavior would be similarly affected by a central stimulant drug, and, conversely, increased by a depressant. While the second expectation was confirmed, the first was not: Not only was there no strain difference, but there was no suggestion of a drug–strain interaction either, hence there is little of pharmacogenetic interest here. Similarly, Watson (1960) using only the "autonomic level" found evidence suggestive of a differentially greater response of the strains' rearing activity during exploration of a novel environment to ephedrine or methylpentynol, with the MNR decreasing and increasing, respectively. Broadhurst *et al.* (1959) failed to confirm this suggestion using the full fourfold pattern of central and autonomic stimulants and depressants and investigating the effect on the various indices provided by the open-field test. Walking activity as measured by ambulation was the only one affected, but by pipradrol only, and there was no interaction with strain.

Perhaps the most thoroughgoing application of the paradigm was that of Singh (1961; Singh and Eysenck, 1960) on the effect of drugs on the development of the conditioned emotional response (CER)—conditioned suppression of lever pressing for water in a Skinner box occasioned by a signal previously associated with shock. In addition to the four drugs noted above, he used combinations of the two "depressants" and the two

TABLE VII

Pharmacology and Psychogenetic Selection: The Maudsley Rat Strains

Reference	Treatment	Measure	Outcome	Remarks
Watson (1960)	Ephedrine and methylpentynol	Rearing	MNR more responsive	
Broadhurst et al. (1959)	Pipradrol, amobarbital, ephedrine and methylpentynol	Open-field test	Pipradrol increased ambulation	
Singh (1961), Singh and Eysenck (1960)	Pipradrol, amobarbital, ephedrine, and methylpentynol	Conditioned suppression of bar pressing	MR more responsive to ephedrine, alone and with pipradrol	
Gupta and Gregory (1967), Holland and Gupta (1967)	Amphetamine, amobarbital, and methylpentynol and combinations	Rearing	Amphetamine increased	
Gregory et al. (1967)	Amphetamine, amobarbital, epinephrine, and methylpentynol	Activity	Amphetamine increased	Same experiment?
Gupta and Holland (1969a,b)	Amphetamine, amobarbital, epinephrine, and methylpentynol	Escape-avoidance conditioning	MR increased with methylpentynol: significant drug-strain interaction	
Gupta and Holland (1972)	Amphetamine and methylpentynol combinations	Open field, rearing, and escape-avoidance conditioning	Amphetamine depressed MRs at high doses	
Garg and Holland (1967, 1968a,b)	Pentobarbital and picrotoxin or nicotine, 2 min after	Hebb–Williams maze, retention	MNR more responsive to stimulants?	Reports unclear
Garg (1969b)	Pentobarbital and picrotoxin or nicotine, 2 min after	Rearing	MNR increase more to stimulants?	Report unclear
Powell (1967), Martin and Powell, (1970)	Amylobarbital	Escape-avoidance conditioning	No interaction	
Garg (1970)	Picrotoxin	Hebb–Williams maze, errors and time	No interaction	

Powell and Hopper (1971)	Amphetamine	Escape-avoidance conditioning	No interaction	
Satinder (1971)	Amphetamine, 30 min before	Escape-avoidance conditioning	No interaction	
Satinder (1971)	Caffeine, 30 min before	Escape-avoidance conditioning	MR increased avoidance more	
Satinder (1972b)	Amphetamine, 30 min before	Intertrial activity, punished	Interaction in avoidance but not intertrial crossing	
Easterbrook (in Broadhurst, 1964)	Injected alcohol	Learning panel push	MR improved	
Powell (1970)	Injected alcohol	T-maze reversal learning	Fewer MR reversals. No interaction	
Broadhurst and Wallgren (1964)	Injected alcohol	Escape-avoidance conditioning	n.s. effect	
Brewster (1968, 1969, 1972)	Alcohol preference	7 different concentrations	Inconsistent findings	F_1, included
Satinder (1972a, 1975)	Alcohol preference	3 different concentrations	MR more, also increased age preference	
Drewek and Broadhurst (1978)	Alcohol preference	6 different concentrations	Both prefer, MR extreme	Sex difference
		Sleep time	n.s. difference	
Keehn (1972)	Trihexiphenidyl	Suppression of schedule-induced alcohol drinking	MNR higher response	
Broadhurst (1964)	Reserpine	Escape-avoidance conditioning	MR facilitated. Drug-strain interaction	
Gregory (1968b)	Prenylamine	Open-field ambulation	MR greater decline	
Satinder (1977a)	Morphine	Rearing	n.s. effect	
Katz (in Kumar and Stolerman, 1973)	Morphine	Preference over quinine after habituation	MR showed some preference, MNR aversion	
		Preference	n.s. difference	
Satinder (1976)	Morphine 1–96 hr before	Escape-avoidance conditioning	MR increased performance	
Garg (1969b,c)	Nicotine, 15 min before	Rearing, frequency	MNR increased	
	Nicotine, 15 min before	Rearing, duration	n.s. effect	
Wraight et al. (1967)	Nicotine, immediately or 5 min after	Underwater Y-maze	n.s. effects	

TABLE VIII
Fourfold Classification of Drugs[a]

Site of action in nervous system	Stimulant	Depressant
Central	Pipradrol (Amphetamine) (Picrotoxin) (Nicotine)	Amylobarbitone (Amobarbital sodium) (Pentobarbital sodium)
Autonomic	Ephedrine	Chlorpromazine (Methylpentynol)

[a]Adapted from Singh (1961): See text.

"stimulants" as well as, in the second study, investigating drug antagonism by means of a graded series of doses of one given in combination with a standard of the other. This comparison was, however, restricted to the two "central" drugs, pipradrol and amylobarbitone. The first study, though marred by the absence of a placebo control against which the change in the bar pressing could be evaluated, and by the failure to distinguish a within-subjects (trials) component from the between-subjects components in the ANOVA, is nevertheless full of interest. For the present purposes it is sufficient to note that the reactive (MR) rats showed a significantly greater sensitivity, as seen by their larger decrements in bar pressing, to the action of ephedrine alone and in combination with pipradrol, than did the nonreactives (MNR). Comparisons of drug effects within the strains were interpreted as supporting this finding. The drug antagonisms were achieved by double injections, and five doses of pipradrol ranging from 2.5 to 40.0 mg/kg were combined with a standard 15 mg/kg of amylobarbitone, whereas five of amylobarbitone (3.75–60 mg/kg) were pitted against the standard of 10 mg/kg of pipradrol. The two standards, of course, were included in combination as center points in the two progressions, and separately as controls, which also included a placebo group. The findings may be summarized by noting that the MR strain again displayed a sensitivity to pipradrol greater than that of the MNR strain, though the two largest doses failed to potentiate the suppression of behavior to the extent that smaller ones did, which the authors compare to a Pavlovian "paradoxical effect." The nonreactives, on the other hand, were found to be more generally responsive to the effects of amylobarbitone (Singh and Eysenck, 1960).

Gupta and Gregory (1967) adopted the design of Singh, including the absence of a placebo control, but extended it to include the effect on rearing of all possible combinations of the four drugs used: amphetamine sulfate, sodium amytal, adrenaline (epinephrine), and methylpentynol. Rearing was measured by capacitance changes in the manner previously described. No strain differences were found in the only effect detected, that of increased rearing attributable to amphetamine. Holland and Gupta (1967) added a placebo group to the same four drugs, no longer in combination but in three increasing dosages over seven days of testing in the rearing apparatus, but once again strain differences were without effect on the response to amphetamine (increase in rearing) and to methylpentynol (decrease). Gregory *et al.* (1967) reported an experiment using precisely the same design and drugs, and, possibly, even the same subjects, to measure the effect on activity in an experimental cage, reporting precisely the same outcome.

Extending the design to five doses of the same four drugs as before, but now administered separately to different animals before 44 trials of two-way avoidance conditioning, required a large number of subjects —200—but yielded greater precision of outcome (Gupta and Holland, 1969a). The drug–strain interaction was fully significant, but was not further modified by dose level. The major constituent of this interaction appears to have been the sensitivity of the MR (reactive) strain to the effects of methylpentynol, which caused a marked increase in successful avoidances.* The effect of amphetamine, while significant, was less pronounced and was, moreover, common to both strains. Intertrial crossings in this experiment, reported separately (Gupta and Holland, 1969b), fairly faithfully reproduced the substantive findings relating to conditioned response acquisition.

A multisituational approach was adopted by Gupta and Holland (1972) in an experiment in which three tests were employed—the open-field test, the rearing cylinder, and two-way avoidance conditioning—but only two drugs were used, amphetamine and methylpentynol, though the effect of the combination of the four progressive doses of each drug was also assayed. The dosages used were 1 + 30 (amphetamine + methylpentynol), 2 + 50, 3 + 70, and 4 + 90 mg/kg. Defecation in the open field was not reported for unspecified reasons, but the ambulation score showed a significant interaction of drug effects with strain, as did the rearing score and one

---

*The reliance that can be placed on this finding is rendered dubious by the observation that the values of the avoidance scores for the various dosage levels of methylpentynol, which can be read off from the authors' Figure 2, together with the placebo value, appear very similar though not identical to those that can be derived from Table 2 and Figure 2 of Holland and Gupta (1966), an earlier and apparently different experiment using methylpentynol only in six rather than five dose levels on rats of the same Maudsley strains but reportedly of a different generation (S_{28} rather than S_{26} and S_{27}). The only exception is the value for the lowest dose of the five in the later paper. While citing their earlier paper, the authors do not draw attention to this remarkable congruity of findings, unusual in behavioral work.

of the scores from the shuttle box, the intertrial crossing score, but not the avoidance score. Again no effect of dose as such was found to differentiate the strains, except in interaction with drug treatments on the avoidance scores, for which the first-order interaction was significant. This complex effect appears to have arisen because of the differential sensitivity of the MR and MNR rats not to the drugs in combination, where the second dosage level produced the best response—that is, the greatest number of avoidances—nor to methylpentynol, for which the third (single) dose was most efficacious, but to amphetamine, which generally showed little dose response among the nonreactives. However, at the highest dose amphetamine markedly depressed performance among the reactives in a way reminiscent of Singh and Eysenck's "paradoxical effect" of pipradrol on this same strain's acquisition of conditioned suppression behavior (1960). The absence of a control group again renders impossible comparisons other than relative ones within the experiment. Study of the simple drug–strain interactions for the other three scores analyzed showed no systematic effect of either drug or their combination, though possibly a multivariate analysis of the various measures would have been appropriate and hence, perhaps, revealing.

Garg and Holland (1967) have extended the approach to the study of posttrial administration, in the manner employed for the work on the Roman strains already referred to. However, only "central" drugs were used, but with two of them (picrotoxin in a dose of 1.0 mg/kg and nicotine, 0.8 mg/kg) being opposed to 10.0 mg/kg of pentobarbital sodium. Again the Hebb–Williams maze was used and the drugs injected intraperitoneally after a 2-min feeding, following single daily trials for nine days, 30 days after which a single retention trial was given following the reimposition of food deprivation. The results, part of which, according to internal evidence in the publications concerned, were republished later in no less than two separate papers relating to picrotoxin (Garg and Holland, 1968b) and pentobarbital sodium (Garg and Holland, 1968a), and will not be referred to again, show that there are significant drug–strain interactions for error scores but not time scores in the ANOVAs of the learning–phase data and for both scores in the retention data. The first interaction additionally involves days (trials) but the data are not presented in such a way as to enable an appraisal of the contribution of strain differences in any of them. The most that can be said is that there appears to be some facilitatory effect of both picrotoxin and of nicotine on the maze learning and that these effects were larger in the nonreactive strain than in the reactive strain.

Garg (1969b) used the same three drugs and possibly the same animals as some of those multiply reported on above, now some 40–50 days older, to assess the effect of the same doses given before four successive daily tests of rearing. Frequency but not duration measures gave a drug–strain interaction that, though once again difficult to interpret from the details given, nevertheless suggests a greater increase among the nonreactives to both nicotine and picrotoxin; the latter drug had no influence on the reactives. Both strains' performance was depressed, as compared with the placebo controls, by pentobarbital sodium.

Studies of single-drug administration using the Maudsley strains as subjects will now be reviewed. In most cases the drug used corresponds to one that has been used in at least one of the studies noticed already, and in some cases supplements what has gone before. Thus Garg (1970) reports further on the study of consolidation in which picrotoxin was used after each learning trial in the Hebb–Williams maze, this time including an additional variable, hunger drive. Neither error nor time scores show a significant interaction in the ANOVAs presented. Broadhurst (1964) informally reported a significant interaction between strain and reserpine, injected intraperitoneally at three dose levels before two-way avoidance conditioning, with some facilitation of the MRs' acquisition as compared with a placebo. Powell (1967), Martin and Powell (1970), Powell and Hopper (1971), and Morrison (1969) report from other laboratories on the use of the strains, the former group inquiring into the effects of amylobarbital sodium and amphetamine on two-way avoidance performance. In neither case was a drug–strain interaction found. The number of rats used was probably too small to detect differences in Morrison's study in which doses of 0.1 or 0.4 mg/kg of nicotine were administered immediately prior to 90-min sessions of operant responding, some of which were punished by shock.

Rivaling the Roman strains in volume of work on the same drug, the Maudsleys have been much studied for their responses to nicotine, some examples of which have already been cited. But most of the work has been of the single-drug form, the "four-drug paradigm" having become attenuated in other work of the Maudsley group, as we have seen. Usually the very high intraperitoneal dose of 0.8 mg/kg was used, as with work on the Roman strains, sometimes included in the same reports, in the manner of Garg's (1969c) investigation of its effects on rearing. However, since the data for the Maudsley strains are arguably the same for the drug group, though probably not for the distilled water controls, as those discussed above (Garg, 1969b) despite their limitation to the first 12 min of the four 15-min trials previously reported, they will not be discussed further.

The high dose employed in these studies is probably less liable to introduce artifactual side effects in studies in which it is administered after trials in tests for consolidation, but even in one of these (Wraight *et al.*, 1967) the dose chosen was 0.25 mg/kg on the grounds that a dose of as little as 0.5 could "lead to debility," though possibly accentuated in this case by the rather more arduous task required of the subjects. This was underwater swimming, the motivation being air deprivation until escape to the surface was achieved, the route lying through an underwater Y-maze with a light discrimination to indicate the correct route. Injections were made either immediately after the five massed trials given daily, or 5 min later. No treatment or treatment × strain effects were detected. In experimentation on posttrial injections in the Hebb–Williams maze, the results of which have already been noted for the Roman strains, Garg and Holland (1969) throw no more light on the findings for the Maudsleys. Indeed, confusion is increased when it is observed that the lower panel of their Figure 2, though not cited in the text but captioned as referring to the data from all four strains, gives the same data as Figure 1 in another paper (Garg and Holland, 1968a), where only the MR and MNR were used as subjects! Since in neither case do the strain differences interact with the nicotine treatment, we can perhaps most charitably pass on without concentrating too much on the problems created by this style of data reporting.

The effects of d-amphetamine sulfate and caffeine on escape-avoidance conditioning were investigated by Satinder (1971) in the context of the results from the Roman strains discussed earlier. The reactive strain showed a clear response to amphetamine and to caffeine, as seen in the increase in number of avoidances, whereas the nonreactives did not. The strains did not differ in their response latencies nor in intertrial activity under amphetamine, which caused both to increase.

In the related study on punished intertrial crossings (Satinder, 1972b), it was found that the punishment again affected the drug–strain interaction in that it differentially depressed the avoidance responding of the MNR strain only, the MRs showing augmentation of responding under amphetamine, irrespective of the additional environmental variation. But the other phenotype examined, intertrial crossing, was minimally affected. In considering these interesting findings it must, however, be noted that the strains did not differ in the acquisition of two-way avoidance conditioned responses, a result at variance with several other reports in the literature [see Broadhurst (1975) for summary].

Prenylamine was also used by Gregory (1968b) in studying both of the Maudsley strains in an investigation paralleling his use of it with one of the Roman strains, as discussed earlier in this chapter. Intraperitoneal injection of 20 mg/kg 3 hr before retesting in the open field caused male rats to respond differentially, the reactive (MR) group showing a greater decline in ambulation. Rearing, however, showed no comparably significant drug–strain interaction.

The effects of alcohol on learning have also been investigated in the

Maudsley strains. Easterbrook reports data (in Broadhurst, 1964) that suggest that oral administration of 1.0 or of 0.5 g/kg (especially) improves the performance of the reactive strain but not the nonreactive strain in a task involving pushing a panel to escape shock, and Powell (1970) injected ethanol (2.4 g/kg) or placebo intraperitoneally before daily trials in a T-maze in which the motivation was also escape from shock to an electrically insulated goal box. Reversal learning to the previously negative, blocked side of the maze was now instituted with the appropriate control for state dependence, that is, the drug condition was now imposed on half the previous saline control subjects and dropped for half the previous drug group, thus giving eight groups, four within each strain, for which comparisons can be made. However, while a marked strain difference (fewer MR reversal errors) was found, no drug–strain interactions, either during the training or during the reversal phase were detected.

This interesting study raises the question of the most appropriate way to measure drug phenotypes in pharmacogenetic investigations. The view taken throughout this review has been to regard the response to a drug as a phenotype in its own right and probably best defined as the difference between performance of drugged and nondrugged subjects. Comparison in this respect of different subjects yields a treatment effect as, for example, might be the case in the study of early environmental experience in which one group is subjected to infantile stimulation and another not so treated. This treatment effect or phenotype in its own right may then itself be shown to vary with strain, giving rise to a treatment–strain interaction, which can be investigated and defined rather precisely in terms of genotype–environment interaction and the genetic architecture subserving it elucidated. The drug–strain interaction is thus merely the phenotypic expression of a possible genotype–environment interaction. But how does state dependence fit into such a schema? The variation among control groups in such a paradigm, that is the drug–drug and the no-drug–no-drug groups, contributes to the drug (treatment) phenotype when intergroup comparisons are made. But when *intra*group comparisons are made, uncontrolled or microenvironmental aspects are presumably also involved, such as the effect of double exposure to the measuring environment. Comparisons within the experimental groups, that is, the drug–no-drug and the no-drug–drug treatment in a typical state-dependence design, can also measure the drug response phenotype as such, the second more obviously than the first. But the whole of this analysis is of course complicated by the test–retest factor mentioned and, worse still, by any learning test differences that may be observed and that inevitably result in distortions. These, however, are inherent in state-dependence designs (Overton, 1973, 1974; Bliss, 1974;

Wright, 1974) and are not peculiar in any way to an analysis into which genetic variables enter in the shape of subjects of different genetic backgrounds (strains and their crosses).

Such complications hardly occur in an analysis of the effect of alcohol on the acquisition by the Maudsley strains of two-way avoidance conditioning (Broadhurst and Wallgren, 1964) since the small to moderate doses (ranging from 0.25 to 2.0 g/kg) injected before a single session of 30 trials had no discernible effect on learning in either strain, only the highest doses being noteworthy as causing an increase in activity.

As was the case with nicotine, so with preference phenotypes, and the Maudsley strains have been used as widely as the Roman, again often combined in the same research. Brewster (1969) studied their preference for a wide range of 7 different concentrations of alcohol from 0.0008% to the more usual 7.9% (wt./vol.). At one of the lowest levels (0.008%) the MNR group was higher than the MR group for intake but not for preference, and at another level (0.08%) the converse was true both for strain and measure. No other differences were significant until the 3.9% and 7.9% levels were compared, at which the reactive subjects assigned to these choices between ethanol and water showed clearly greater consumption than the nonreactives, both in preference and intake measures. But this finding did not stand up to replication, at least in part, since animals from later generations of the selection experiment, when offered 3.9% concentration as the choice, gave strong indications that the MNR group was now the higher preference strain. This reversal was confirmed in another study, reported by Brewster in 1968 and again in 1972. In it, rats from the same generation (and possibly the same individuals) were crossed to provide an F_1 to enable one of the rare genetic analyses of pharmacological phenotypes* undertaken on material derived from psychogenetic selection experiments, and data were reported on all four generations (parentals and the two reciprocal F_1s). The reciprocal crosses allowed a test of the possibility of maternal effects on the preference and intake phenotypes, and were shown to be negligible. This is perhaps the most satisfactory part of the analysis, since a breeding design as restricted as this, however novel in this field, allows little scope for detailed biometrical genetical analysis. What evidence there is, however, points to a substantial additive genetic component of the variation in both phenotypes, with dominance towards the higher scoring parental strain, the MNR in this case, especially with respect to intake scores.

These findings must be treated with caution, however, in view of the discrepancies over the relative standing of the two parental strains revealed in Brewster's work, and this caution is reinforced by a consideration of

*Though see footnote on page 7.

Satinder's extensive findings (1972*a*, 1975) on these same strains, along with those for the three Roman strains. He reports throughout that it is the Maudsley reactives and not the nonreactives which are the higher consuming strain at the 3.9%, 7.9%, and 15.8% (wt./vol.) concentration levels used, and significantly so at the first two. Additionally, the MRs showed the greatest increase, and indeed the only significant one among the five strains studied, in intake of alcohol during the sustained period of forced consumption, though it was also the only one to show a significant decrease in intake after the week of alcohol deprivation. In contrast, the MNR group showed little change during forced consumption but did show an increase after deprivation, the significance of which was not mentioned in the report, though it was of the order of that for the RHA strain, which was significant. It is perhaps noteworthy that this result was the only report in Satinder's studies of the MNR showing higher consumption than the MRs, which they demonstrated in two of Brewster's three experiments using these selected strains. In the study of the effect of food deprivation on preference also reported by Satinder (1972*a,b*), the MR rats consistently consumed larger amounts of alcohol than the MNRs, perhaps accounting for their insensitivity to the changes introduced in dietary regimen, to which the lower consuming nonreactive rats responded significantly on both of the occasions on which it was introduced. In the further work on age differences as determinants of consumption (Satinder, 1975), the reactive strain increased in preference with age while the nonreactives did not. At both the ages studied (commencing at 28 and 105 days of age), the reactives usually consumed more than the nonreactives, though this was not true for all the numerous concentrations utilized, ranging from 0.2% to 50% (wt./vol.), but there does not seem to be any pattern to the exceptions at the two ages that would explain Brewster's conflicting results. In attempting to account for these findings, he had invoked age differences among his subjects (1969). The extended Experiment 2 of Satinder again showed the MR group as more alcohol prone, in that, for example, it was the only one of the five strains in which the subgroup allowed water did not consume more alcohol in the periodic preference tests than the group forced to drink alcohol, thus showing that alcohol preference was strong in this strain and little affected by chronic ingestion.

Drewek and Broadhurst's work (1978) on strain difference in alcohol preference can be usefully cited once again, since the Maudsley strains were included among those studied using the three-bottle two-choice technique. Both the MR and MNR strains show sustained, though not markedly high, preference ratios, but the most striking feature of the data was the marked increase in the intake and in calorie contribution measures with increasing concentration. Indeed, the MR strain, which displayed this tendency to a greater extent than the MNR, was shown to have reached an average daily intake of 8.5 g/kg/day when the final (12% wt./vol.) concentration was reached—about the level of Eriksson's AA strain after 16 generations of selection (Eriksson, 1971*b*; see Chapter 3). Females were even more extreme than the males, a general finding for this measure for almost all values of alcohol concentration offered in the test solutions. Once again, no strain differences in sleep times in response to injected alcohol were found.

As a final appendage to the work on alcohol preference in the Maudsley strains, mention may be made of Keehn's work (1972) on operant schedule-induced drinking of alcohol and its suppression by trihexiphenidyl. The numbers of subjects used were small but the tendency was for the *nonreactives* to have a higher intake; all subjects, however, responded equally to the antidipsogenic compound.

Moving on to work on morphine (Satinder, 1977*a*), the results of the 50-day regimen imposed in the way previously discussed showed that the Maudsley strains differ in the development of their response to increasing forced intake of morphine. The reactives (MR) showed some development of preference, though not quite so markedly as the Roman high-avoidance strain, whereas the nonreactives evidenced some aversion. The forced abstinence test gave results similar to those for the Roman strains, that is, there was no tendency among either to respond with enhanced intake. In the quinine control tests also reported by Satinder (1977*a*) the MR strain was confirmed as not far below the Roman strains in the development of preference just as was the MNR, a nonpreferring strain. Thus these strains showed consistent differences throughout Satinder's work. Results for these strains on the development of morphine dependence were also informally reported by Katz (in Kumar and Stolerman, 1973), who recorded no very clear differences between them.

Application of the increasing series of doses of morphine, as used by Satinder (1976) with the Roman selection strains, showed that among the Maudsley strains the effect on two-way escape–avoidance conditioning was similarly to increase the performance of the lower-scoring strain, in this case the MR rats, so that at the 1-hr interval after the last of the injections they returned higher avoidance scores than the MNR group, again without any significant difference in intertrial crossing activity. After longer time intervals the advantage is less apparent amid the general decline in all scores, as previously reported. More weight can be given to this finding of facilitation by morphine since both control groups show the usual superiority of the nonreactive MNR strain in avoidance measures, though it should be noted that as many as half of the twelve MR strain tested succumbed, and it is not clear what effect if any these fatalities and the consequent loss of data had on the analyses presented.

Our survey of psychopharmacological work on the Maudsley strains allows few definite conclusions to be drawn from it. Despite a considerable investment of time, effort, and subjects—though not so much as the multiple reporting that seems to have characterized the literature on these topics would lead the casual reader to believe—the outcome is relatively meager and my impression— albeit, doubtless, a biased one as the founder of the strains in question—is of opportunities missed. The reliable definition of interstrain differences in drug response, without which no satisfactory genetic analysis is possible, has hardly begun, and it is perhaps ironic that the most sophisticated attempt to do so was on the basis of the shifting sands of the difference in alcohol preference between the strains, now reversed from that assumed on the basis of his results by Brewster. Indeed, it is in this connection perhaps that some glimmers of light are to be seen, since Satinder's and Drewek and Broadhurst's evidence now rather clearly points to a reasonably definite and robustly reliable difference between the strains in favor of a higher preference among the Maudsley reactives, which clearly merits further study.

What I have termed the "four-drug paradigm" played an important part in studies using these strains, and in initiating their pharmacogenetic study. Its early promise was not, however, sustained, and the caveats and cautions of its earliest enunciators such as Singh were in the end lost sight of, as was, apparently, the whole purpose of contrasting drug actions. It is not surprising that in this climate of opinion, comprehension of the possibilities as well as the complexities of the genetic analysis of drug actions as a phenotype failed to develop as might have been hoped.

This also brings us toward the end of our consideration of the pharmacogenetics of strains derived from behavioral selection experiments, with a few exceptions, summarized in Table IX. The first relates to work done by Lát and his collaborators using rats bidirectionally selected for what is termed "non-specific excitation level" (Lát and Gollová-Hémon, 1969) and which consists of a phenotype defined in terms of the amount of vertical rearing recorded in an automatic electrocapacitance device. Few details of the kind and degree of genetic selection practiced are available: One report (Lát and Gollová, 1964) that mentions the S_5 and S_6 generations describes observations of exploratory activity of this type taken from them after three doses of amphetamine of 0.25, 2.0, and 5.0 mg/kg, which interacted differentially with strain. It was claimed that "The doses exerting maximal effect are lower in both groups of animals with extremely low and high innate levels of excitability than with medium excitable animals" (p. 201), which suggests that comparison was made with a third, unselected strain, but no further details were given in this rather brief report.

Similar obscurity surrounds the provenance of rats used by Votava and

TABLE IX

Pharmacology and Psychogenetic Selection: Various Strains of Rat, Mouse, and Dog

Reference	Species	Selection	Generation	Treatment	Measure	Outcome	Remarks
Lát and Gollová (1964)	Rat	Bidirectional, "nonspecific excitation level"	S_5, S_6	Amphetamine 0.25, 2.0, and 5.0 mg/kg	Vertical rearing, automatically recorded	Drug–strain interaction	? Unselected strain assessed. Details lacking
Votava and Soušková (1965)	Rat	Bidirectional, excitability		Chlorpromazine, 1.0 and 2.0 mg/kg Chlorprothixene, 1.0 and 2.0 mg/kg Chlorprohepta-triene, 5.0 and 9.5 mg/kg subcutaneous Other drugs (Soušková and Benešová, 1963)	Vertical rearing, manually recorded in 10 min period 1 hr after injection	Drug–strain interaction. High excitables more drug susceptible	
Müller-Calgan et al. (1973)	Rat	Bidirectional, escape-avoidance conditioning	S_{12}–S_{16}	Amphetamine 2.0 mg/kg Diazepam 1.0 mg/kg	Pain sensitivity (observational)	No strain differences Sex-strain interaction	
Masur et al. (1975)	Rat	Bidirectional, food competition success LRS and WRS strains	S_5	Apomorphine 1.0 mg/kg dopa 100, 150, 200 mg/kg intraperitoneally	Pushing opponent down tube	Drugs increased success of LRS vs. undrugged WRS	Design not suited to show drug-strain interaction
Lagerspetz and Lagerspetz (1971)	Mouse	Aggression, TA and TNA strains		d-amphetamine	LD_{50} values	No interaction. Isolate/group rearing interacted with strain (increased TA aggression)	Not a behavioral measure
van Abeelen (1974)	Mouse	Rearing frequency, SRH and SRL strains	S_{19}	Scopolamine	Rearing and activity	SRH rearing and activity reduced	

Reference	Species	Subjects	S	Drug	Activity	Drug–strain interaction	Strain differences abolished
van Abeelen et al. (1975)	Mouse		S_{19}	Scopolamine methylbromide, 1.0 and 2.0 μg. Intracranial hippocampal injection		Drug–strain interaction. SRH decreased	Strain differences abolished
Murphree (1972)	Dog	Timidity, E and A strains	S_3	Anxiolytics	Observation and rating of timidity. Also bar-press operant task	Improved performance for E strain	
Murphree et al. (1974a)	Dog	E strain	S_3	Chlordiazepoxide		Improvement continued after drug termination. Improvement easily disrupted	
Angel et al. (1974)	Dog	E and A dogs		Chlordiazepoxide, 1.75, 2.0, 3.75, and 5.0 mg/kg	Bar-press operant task	Increased dose improved E performance to level of A strain (unaffected by drug). Drug–strain interaction	
				Amphetamine or cocaine (0.25 and 0.50 mg/kg) 2 hr after chlordiazepoxide		Drug–strain interaction again. A strain less disrupted than E	Lack of statistical test
Murphree et al. (1974b)	Dog	E strain and catahoulas		Alcohol	Operant task		Inappropriate comparison
De Luca et al. (1974)	Dog	Matched pairs E and A		Tranylcypromine after tryptophan loading	Behavioral and biochemical	No differences found	
Newton et al. (1976)	Dog			Methylphenidate, 0.5 mg/kg	Physiological indices of cardiac and respiratory function	E showed delay of return to baseline after methylphenidate depression	

Soušková (1965) in a study in which one generation of selection for the two extremes of excitability, defined as before but recorded manually, and for a medium-excitable group was apparently involved. Three drugs, chlorpromazine, chlorprothixene (both in 1.0 and 2.0 mg/kg doses), and chlorproheptatriene (5.0 and 9.5 mg/kg) were used and there was some differential response of the strains in terms of the amount of activity observed during 10 min of observation, 1 hr after subcutaneous injection. The high-excitable strain proved to be generally more susceptible. Results for other drugs were reported in abstract (Soušková and Benešová, 1963).*

Another selection for escape–avoidance conditioning in rats as in the Roman strains was reported by Müller-Calgan and Schorscher (1973) to have reached generations S_{14} and S_{16} in the (replicated) high strains, and S_{12} and S_{15} in the low. Crossbreeding at the S_5 generation gave some suggestions of a maternal effect in the second filial generation (F_2). Müller-Calgan et al. (1973) noted the absence of strain differences in response to amphetamine (2.0 mg/kg) and diazepam (1.0 mg/kg), and in pain sensitivity, all, however, assessed by observational techniques. More prominent were sex differences, which interacted in various ways with the drugs given.

A bidirectional selection experiment for winning or losing in a food-seeking competition, in the manner described earlier (see Chapter 2), was reported by Masur and Benedito (1974a) to have reached the S_5 generation with appreciable differentiation between the strains. There was no correlated response to the behavioral selection in body weight changes and the institution of a partial (postnatal) control for maternal effects by the routine use of foster mothers. The effects of pharmacological manipulation of the behavior of one only of the two strains, the selected *loser* strain or LRS, in competition with undrugged subjects from the *winner* or WRS strain was reported by Masur et al. (1975). However, the structure of the experiment, as described, obviously precludes any possibility of drug–strain interaction. To observe such interaction, competition between *both* strains under drug conditions or possibly each separately against the same neutral strain would be required. Nevertheless, it is worth noting that the effects of apomorphine (1.0 mg/kg) or of dopa (1-dihydroxyphenylalanine-methylester hydrochloride) (100, 150, and 200 mg/kg) given intraperitoneally to males and to females, respectively, of the loser strain 10 min before contests with rats of the same sexes of the winner strain, not

---

*Equally difficult to interpret is a mention by Boissier et al. (1976) of the "interbreeding" of two strains of rats for high and low speed of defecation in a nonstandard form of open-field test. While no fewer than five generations were reported to have been bred, it is not clear if genetical selection as properly understood had been practiced and consequently it is not surprising that progress towards the establishment of divergent phenotypes for use in a psychopharmacological context has been disappointing.

medicated, was to increase, usually significantly, the number of contests won by pushing the opponent back along the narrow tube.

A brief report by Lagerspetz and Lagerspetz (1971) deals with the toxic effects of *d*-amphetamine on their strains not of rats but of mice selectively bred for high and low aggressivity (TA for *T*urku *a*ggressive and TNA for *T*urku *n*onaggressive, respectively). No differences in LD_{50} values were found, so there is no evidence of drug–strain interaction and the response is hardly a behavioral one in any case, but it is perhaps of interest that an experiential variable (being reared in isolation as opposed to groups of five or more) interacted with strain to increase the aggressiveness of the TA mice, while not affecting their susceptibility to amphetamine. Mention may also be made of a brief reference by Whitney *et al.* (1970) to mice from an early stage of De Fries' and Hegmann's bidirectional selection for open-field activity (1970) in relation to alcohol preference. These results will be considered later (see Section 9.1).

Van Abeelen (1970) described the establishment by selective breeding based on an F_2 cross derived from C57BL/6J and DBA/2J inbred strains of mice of two strains differentiated with respect to their rearing frequency as measured by counting the number of vertical excursions made during 15 min in an empty observation cage. At generations prior to S_{19} these SRH and SRL mice (*S*-rearing *h*igh and *l*ow) were shown to differ with respect to whole-brain acetylcholinesterase, the SRH generally giving significantly lower values than the SRL (van Abeelen, 1974). Modification of their behavior was then achieved by using the anticholinergic scopolamine, injected peripherally, which, especially at low doses, lowered the rearing and other exploratory activity of the high (SRH) strain. To test if the cholinergic mechanism believed to facilitate exploration is located centrally or peripherally, van Abeelen *et al.* (1975) used the quaternary congener of scopolamine, scopolamine methylbromide, a compound previously shown not to affect such behavior in inbred mice when injected peripherally (van Abeelen *et al.*, 1971; see Chapter 7) and hence unlikely to pass the blood–brain barrier readily. This drug was injected intracranially into mice of the S_{19} generation, directly into the hippocampus, the area hypothesized to be the location of the cholinergic mechanism governing exploratory activity. The results unequivocally supported the hypothesis in that the SRH strain decreased their activity markedly, whereas the low (SRL) increased theirs slightly, so that at the higher of the two doses used (1.0 and 2.0 μg) the significant difference between them was abolished.

Finally, response to drugs has been reported in the context of a further selection experiment in yet another species, the dog. Murphree and Dykman [1965; see Dykman *et al.* (1969) for review] began, in 1960 in Arkansas, to breed two strains of pointer dogs: one, the E strain showing timidity and fearfulness, especially toward humans, and the other, the A strain, being essentially normal in this respect. The parental population was relatively loosely defined, but was drawn from different samples of the pointer breed. The phenotype was measured using a series of relatively simple, observational tests in which ratings for fearfulness showed good reliability. Numbers are necessarily small with an animal as expensive to rear and maintain as the dog but by the third generation (Murphree *et al.*, 1967*a*) good separation had been achieved between the two lines. Crossbred subjects were shown (Murphree *et al.*, 1969) to display potence, that is, phenotypic dominance, for stability rather than fearfulness at all ages studied between 2 and 12 months of life, and the absence of phenotypic differences between such crossbred dogs reared by either timid E strain mothers or by normal A strain ones was taken to indicate the absence of important maternal effects (Murphree and Newton, 1971), though more extensive tests involving cross-fostering would be needed to establish this point unequivocally (see discussion in Section 9.1). Parent–offspring correlations are reported (Murphree, 1973), but not separately for each strain, so that their use in analyzing the progress of selection is minimal.

This then was the material in which the psychopharmacological studies were undertaken, largely, one gets the impression, in the context of the study of various procedures that might be used to "normalize" the E strain subjects, including various techniques of canine behavior modification, among them desensitization (McBryde and Murphree, 1974). An early experiment (Murphree, 1972) was apparently restricted to subjects of the E strain who showed, in response to medication with various anxiolytics, an improved performance in the rating scales mentioned above and in an operant conditioning task adapted for dogs (Murphree *et al.*, 1967*b*). In response to chlordiazepoxide, though improvement due to this treatment was seen in other contexts, it was only observed to continue with some subjects after the termination of medication and was easily disturbed, so that the typical fearful behavior including inactivity and failure to bar press was reinstated (Murphree *et al.*, 1974*a*).

In subsequent work in which both strains were used, thus allowing the possibility of the detection of a drug–strain interaction, Angel *et al.* (1974) used four dogs from each of the two strains in the bar-pressing task after having demonstrated that there was no significant difference in the rate of clearance of chlordiazepoxide between them. Increasing intravenous doses of the drug (1.75, 2.00, and 3.75 mg/kg), though not given in that order, were necessary to establish and maintain the operant response for food on a CRF schedule for dogs of the E strain, and the effect of 5 mg/kg/day was quite dramatic. First, it restored their performance to a level indistinguishable from that of the A strain, which was essentially unchanged throughout, and second, on withdrawal caused it to fall to a premedication level. In this way a clear drug–strain interaction on the phenotype was demonstrated. Further work in which the effect of chlordiazepoxide was antagonized by either amphetamine or cocaine, both given in dosages of 0.25 or 0.50 mg/kg 2 hr after either 1.75 or 4.0 mg/kg of chlordiazepoxide, also yielded data suggestive of such an interaction. The stable A strain dogs showed less marked disruption of bar pressing than did the E strain, though the absence of statistical evaluation of the data renders this conclusion less clear-cut than in the former case mentioned above. This theme is also apparent in subsequent work (Murphree *et al.*, 1974*b*) in which the effect of a large number of drugs including alcohol was assessed on the operant task. But the possibility of an effective comparison with implications for genetic interpretation of the drug response was lessened by the use, for comparison purposes with the selected E strain, of not the A strain of pointers but another breed of dog, catahoulas, who themselves showed some degree of disturbance, though less marked than the E strain. In this connection it should be pointed out that the importation into a selection experiment of genetic stocks not represented in the original parental population must inevitably attenuate the crispness of any possible comparison between strains established by directional selection. There is some suggestion that such a procedure had already occurred in the Arkansas experiment (Murphree, 1973) but from within the pointer breed, which would presumably represent a population relatively well defined genetically.

To conclude, DeLuca *et al.* (1974) in some of their experiments used a monoamine oxidase inhibitor, tranylcypromine, after tryptophan loading in matched pairs of dogs from the two strains in order to assess behavioral and biochemical differences. No differences were detected with this technique, whereas the use of methylphenidate (Newton *et al.*, 1976) to assess its effects on physiological indices of cardiac function and respiration revealed some differences. The E strain (nervous) subjects showed, for example, a significantly delayed return to baseline heart rate after the depression caused by methylphenidate (0.5 mg/kg).

This coda to the present section of this review perhaps points up the adventitious nature of some of the psychopharmacological work on the various selectively bred strains and the need to integrate adequate genetical analysis with advanced pharmacology.

Chapter 5

Strain Differences I: Amphetamine and Other Stimulants

5.1. Variability of Response

The study of strain differences in the drug responses of nonselected subjects had included other species of laboratory animals than the widely used rat, the range now being extended to, especially, the mouse. This species has long been available in inbred strains in a profusion not evident for the rat, the laboratory animal most favored by psychologists. The reason is that the mouse has been used by workers in the field of cancer research and inbred strains of mice were developed in the interests of uniformity of response to drug and other treatments, including susceptibility to spontaneous carcinomas and response to carcinogens, in a way that was not paralleled for the rat.

The problem of uniformity of drug response has been of some importance in drug assay, and not the least with respect to the psychotropic agents studied by psychopharmacologists. It impinges on the theme of this monograph because it is recognized that part, at least, of the variability encountered in the measurement of drug phenotypes is genetically modulated since it has been noted that animals from long-inbred—and hence genetically uniform—strains were often less consistent in their individual responses than first filial crosses derived from two such strains [see, for example, McLaren and Michie (1956)].

In an interesting example of this effect, Mackintosh (1962) combined the isolation variable, as used by Lagerspetz and Lagerspetz (1971), though extending it to three different sizes of groups, with susceptibility to quinalbarbitone sodium anesthesia. He showed that not only did the two mouse strains used (CE and CBA) differ in the variance of their sleep times in response to a dosage graded for body weight, but that reciprocal F_1 animals had a markedly lower variance than either. Mice housed in pairs showed the lowest variance overall. There is also some suggestion of a maternal effect on variability in that the cross having mothers from the less variable strain (CE) were themselves less variable than those fathered by CEs, but in the absence of the group means and of information about how the filial crosses were reared, this finding remains no more than suggestive.

The possible utility of this difference in variability was pointed out as long ago as 1946 by Mather and stems from the fact that animals from an F_1 cross of homozygous strains are also genetically uniform, like their parents. However, the uniformity is of a different kind, being that of a complete heterozygosity—at least for all gene loci at which the parents differ—half of the genetic material being derived from each parent. Now, heterozygous material is often better buffered against environmental pressure than genetic purebreds, hence the greater uniformity of response to the essentially environmental treatment offered by the drug. Herein lies the possible advantage of F_1 hybrids over purebred strains for bioassay.

While this problem is of interest in connection with the topic of this book, it is not central to it since the genetics of variability in drug responsivity as such has entered pharmacogenetics as a technical problem of psychopharmacology, concerned with minimizing that variability rather than analyzing its causation. Consequently, the matter has not been pursued as vigorously as could have been wished and precise explanations are not available. It seems likely, however, that the phenomenon is based on a genotype–environment interaction mechanism, that is, a differential response to environmental pressure mediated through a buffering mechanism of the kind that has been demonstrated to exist in other contexts (e.g., Fulker, 1970).

After this digression on a particular problem we turn, then, to the study of strain differences as such. Here, we encounter a wide-ranging literature bearing on drug–strain interactions, but once again we must remember that the demonstration of a strain difference constitutes no more than presumptive evidence of some degree of genetical determination, and the establishment of its amount and its character is only to be accomplished by genetical techniques, especially cross breeding, which have been relatively rarely used.

Organizationally, we shall proceed as before with consideration being given first to broadly stimulant drugs before turning to depressants and ending with work on alcohol preferences and drugs of dependence. Two further divergences from this progression will, however, be encountered. Both of them relate to particular genetical techniques used in psychopharmacogenetics. The work employing them is relatively limited and best dealt with in a methodological context since it overlaps relatively little with what is discussed elsewhere.

5.2. Amphetamine and Other Stimulants

Response to amphetamine has been widely studied in mouse strains, as may be seen from the numerous entries in summary Table X. Moisset and Welch (1973) used two inbred strains, a black (C57BL/10J) and an albino (BALB/cJ) and showed that the blacks responded substantially more to an intraperitoneal dose of 5 mg/kg of *d*-amphetamine on ambulation activity in seven successive daily open-field tests. A generalized hyperactivity rather than a specific test response was, however, suspected.

As part of a study in which amphetamine was taken as an exemplar of a stimulant drug in the progression sedation–tranquilization–stimulation–convulsion (the others in this progression paradigm being pentobarbital, chlorpromazine, and pentylenetetrazol, respectively), Meier *et al.* (1963) had used the same black and albino mouse strains (though in different sublines—C57BL/6 and BALB/c) as well as two others, DBA/2 and C3H. These four were themselves intended to represent another progression—a continuum of arousal. Activity was measured in a jiggle cage automatically recording any movement of the subject leading to oscillation about a fulcrum, on one occasion after 25 mg/kg of *d*-amphetamine injected intraperitoneally. The C57BL/6 (black) subline was alone in showing an effect of increased activity, which lasted into the second half (15–30 min) of the record: The others showed some transitory increases. A precise rendering of the nature of the drug–strain interaction in these effects is complicated by a saline-injection-induced depression in activity, confirmed by separate tests in only two of the strains (BALB/c and DBA/2).

Satinder *et al.* (1970) also used amphetamine together with chlorpromazine to study their effects on the factor scores of two mouse strains, SWR/J and SJL/J, on a battery of tests of emotional reactivity. The same two doses, 1.0 and 2.0 mg/kg, of each drug were used, and it was found that amphetamine reversed the standing of the two strains in the first factor considered, that interpreted as relating to freezing behavior. Chlorpromazine had no significant effect on this factor, and neither drug affected the other factor, characterized as relating to disorganization of behavior in the subtests of the battery that defined it. The support these findings give to a hypothesis of the relative position of the strains along a continuum of arousal, of the kind suggested by Meier *et al.*, is limited both by the

TABLE X

Psychopharmacogenetic Experiments with Amphetamine and Other Stimulants

Reference	Species (and strain)	Drug	Measure	Outcome	Remarks
Moisset and Welch (1973)	Mice, C57BL/10J, BALB/cJ	Amphetamine	Open-field ambulation	C57BL/10J > BALB/cJ	Generalized activity?
Meier *et al.* (1963)	Mice, C57BL/6, BALB/c, DBA/2, C3H	Amphetamine	Jiggle-cage activity	C57BL/6 increased	
Satinder *et al.* (1970)	Mice, SWR/J, SJL/J	Amphetamine, chlorpromazine	Emotional reactivity factors	Strains reversed n.s. effect	
Scott *et al.* (1971)	Mice, C57BL/6, BALB/c	Amphetamine	Induced fighting	C57BL/6 aggression reduced more	
Lapin (1974)	Mice, C57BL/6, BALB/c, C57BR	Amphetamine	Toxicity Activity and emotional reactivity	C57BL/6 most resistant	
Davis *et al.* (1974)	Mice, C57BL/10J, BALB/cJ	Amphetamine	Aggregation toxicity	BALB/cJ LD_{50} lower	C57BL/10J more stable response
Bovet and Oliverio (1967)	Mice, DBA/2J, C3H/He	Amphetamine	Escape-avoidance conditioning	Amphetamine restored performance	
Richardson *et al.* (1972)	Mice, including C57BL/6J, also deermice, meadow voles	Methamphetamine	Exploratory, social, and aggressive behavior	No drug-strain interaction	

Reference	Species/strains	Drug	Task	Result	Major gene
Werboff et al. (1967)	Mice, C57BL, A/J, DBA/2J, AKR/J, four-way cross	Amphetamine	Water escape	Amphetamine response, no interaction with coat color n.s. effect	pleiotropism
Isaeva and Krasuskii (1961)	Dog	Caffeine	Swim weighted Conditioned reflex disruption	Strong and weak nervous systems identified	
Ginsburg et al. (1976)	Dogs, beagle × (1) coyote, (2) Telomian	Amphetamine, barbiturates	Hyperkinesis	(1) No effect (2) Amphetamine improved, barbiturate not	
Lucas and Scott (1977)	Dogs, beagle × Telomian	Amphetamine	Restraint	Increased, possible maternal effect	Reciprocal cross
Morrison and Stephenson (1973)	Rats, Lister, Lister × Sprague-Dawley	Amphetamine, nicotine	Operant responses	Not evaluated	Numbers small
Beckwith et al. (1974)	Rats, Long-Evans hooded, albinos	Amphetamine	Brightness-discrimination learning	Hooded > albinos	
Barrett et al. (1973)	Rats, Sprague-Dawley, Fischer	Amphetamine, scopolamine	Discriminated escape-avoidance	Increase in Sprague-Dawleys	Drug–strain interaction
Anisman (1975a,c)	Mice, C57BL/6J, DBA/2J, A/J	Amphetamine, scopolamine	Discriminated escape-avoidance	C57BL/6J did not improve; only A/J improved	Drug–strain interaction
Anisman (1976b)	Mice, C57BL/6J, DBA/2J, A/J	Amphetamine, scopolamine	Conventional escape-avoidance	C57 poorer than salines. A/J facilitated by both drugs. DBA disrupted by scopolamine	Drug–strain interaction

(Continued)

TABLE X—Continued

Reference	Species (and strain)	Drug	Measure	Outcome	Remarks
Anisman (1975a)	Mice, C57BL/6J, DBA/2J, A/J	Amphetamine	Inhibitory avoidance	C57BL/6J immune to disruption	
Anisman and Kokkinidis (1975)	Mice, C57BL/6J, DBA/2J, A/J	Amphetamine	Activity in Y-maze	Perseverative effects	
		Amphetamine with or without α-MpT, FLA-63	Activity in Y-maze	Enzyme inhibitors alone effective only in DBA. Amphetamine-induced increase antagonized except in DBA	
Anisman and Cygan (1975)	Mice, C57BL/6J, DBA/2J, A/J	Amphetamine with or without FLA-63	Open-field activity, shock response	Amphetamine-induced increase antagonized only in C57BL/6J	
Anisman et al. (1975)	Mice, C57BL/6J, DBA/2J, A/J	Amphetamine, scopolamine	Open-field activity, shock response	Amphetamine enhanced activity especially after shock. Little effect of scopolamine	Confirmed for scopolamine (Anisman, 1975b)
Oliverio et al. (1966)	Mice, DBA, C3H/He	Scopolamine	Escape-avoidance conditioning	DBA greater increase	
van Abeelen and Strijbosch (1969), van Abeelen (1974)	Mice, C57BL/6, DBA/2 and F_1	Scopolamine, physostigmine	Exploration	Drug-strain interaction No interaction	
Bovet and Oliverio (1973), Oliverio (1974b), Oliverio and Bovet (1975)	Mice, C57BL, DBA, and F_1, C57BL, SEC/1 ReJ and F_1	Amphetamine Scopolamine Physostigmine	Tilt-cage activity	C57BL activity reduced, F_1s vary DBA and F_1 increase n.s. difference	Potence suggested Result for C57BL atypical Not confirmed by Oliverio et al. (1973a)
Lapin (1975)	Mice, DBA, BALB, C57BL/6J, C3H/A SUB	Apomorphine	Ambulation and rearing	Drug-strain interaction	C57BL/6J again distinct from all others

Reference	Strains	Drug	Task	Result	Comments
van Abeelen et al. (1971, 1972)	Mice, C57BL, DBA and cross	Scopolamine, neostigmine	Exploration	Drug-strain interaction	Replicated earlier work Supports central cholinergic facilitation
Remington and Anisman (1976)	Mice, C57BL, DBA, A/J	Amphetamine, scopolamine	Open-field activity of juveniles	Increase (DBAs after 14 days) Increase—age dependent (DBA earlier), i.e., age-strain interaction	Differential maturation of biochemical systems
Morrison and Lee (1968)	Rats, Lister, Wistar Sprague–Dawley	Physostigmine, nicotine	Behavioral phenotypes	Drug-strain interaction	Long-term experiment
Cazala (1976)	Mice, C57BL/6, DBA/2, BALB/c, (all/Or1)	d- and l-Amphetamine	Intensity of intracranial self-stimulation	Drug-strain interaction. Interactions of strain also with isomer and electrode placement. Largest effects in C57BL	
Anisman (1976a)	Mice, A, DBA/2, C57BL/6, and crosses	d-Amphetamine, scopolamine	Open-field activity before and after shock	Activity before and after amphetamine and after shock are responses mediated by different genetic mechanisms	Complete diallel cross

definitive results and the absence of any inbred strains common to the two experiments.

Scott *et al.* (1971) employed the same sublines of C57BL and BALB mice as Meier *et al.* to investigate the effect of amphetamine on fighting. They found that a dose of 10 mg/kg of *d*-amphetamine reduced forced aggression—induced by dangling an intruder mouse into subjects' home territory—in both strains, but only significantly among the blacks, and sought to relate this difference to the differential body temperature response of the two strains to a series of doses ranging from 0.07 to 20.0 mg/kg. At lower levels a sharp decline was observed after 20 min in both strains, whereas above 5.0 the BALB albino strain showed elevated temperatures characteristic of the amphetamine aggregation toxicity effect of Chance [1946: mentioned by Gunn and Gurd (1940); see Thiessen (1964) for review]. Lapin (1974) confirmed the C57BL strain's resistance to toxicity using these same two strains, together with the C57BR, also showing that equitoxic doses of amphetamine increased activity and emotional reactivity least among the C57BL mice. Davis *et al.* (1974) did the same, reporting that while doses as large as 26.0 mg/kg caused little mortality among solitary mice of both strains after 24 hr, among groups of 10 the LD_{50} was significantly lower at 4.1 mg/kg for BALB/cJ mice than for the C57BL/10J used (9.7 mg/kg). But further work on activity after amphetamine and using both additional strains (four) and additional variables (three levels of illumination) gave findings that suggested that drug–strain interactions were present. Their study indicated that their origin lay primarily in the smaller activity response to the drug of the BALB mice as compared with the C57s (and others). Noteworthy in the present context is the instability of response in different experiments of subjects from the former strain, albeit from different colonies, which may be contrasted with a relative stability of ones from the latter, even though from different substrains (C57BL/6 Cum and /10J).

Bovet and Oliverio (1967) were interested in the effect of amphetamine (1.5 mg/kg) in restoring the performance of mice of the DBA/2J and C3H/He strains in escape–avoidance conditioning, after it had declined to low levels (around 3%–6% successful avoidances) at the end of a marathon series of 2500 trials in the shuttle box lasting many hours. This it successfully did, but the differences between the strains in the extent of the improvement also varied according to the amount of training given prior to the marathon, and hence it is not clear if a drug–strain interaction can be deduced from these data.

Three strains of mice were included by Richardson *et al.* (1972) in a comparison of the effects of methamphetamine sulfate on several rodent species, ranging from deer mice to meadow voles (see also Section 7.3). The effects of either a single dose (7.0 mg/kg) or five successive daily doses, increasing geometrically from 3.0 to 48 mg/kg, were observed for 75 min in a large area comprising many interconnecting chambers and starting 15 min after intraperitoneal injection. While differences from controls were detected in the several aspects of exploratory and social, including aggressive, behavior observed, and species varied in the extent of these differences, no marked drug–strain interactions were reported within the group of three mouse strains used, one of which was the C57BL/6J.

Werboff *et al.* (1967) crossed C57BL mice with an albino strain we have not yet encountered in this chapter, A/J, and obtained black F_1 offspring, since the albino or nonpigmented coat color is recessive to all others. Another black F_1 was also generated by crossing DBA/2J mice, phenotypically gray but carrying the major gene for black, with yet another albino strain, the AKR/J. Crossing these two F_1s together allowed Mendelian segregation for coat color in the proportion 2:1:1 (black: brown: albino) and a sample from this four-way cross—so called because four parental strains were involved—was tested in several situations. The purpose was to investigate further the Keeler–King hypothesis (1941) that temperament in rodents is associated, perhaps causally, with the major genes determining coat color (see Wilcock, 1969, for a review). Among the tests used was response to intraperitoneal doses of *d*-amphetamine of 5, 10, or 20 mg/kg given 1 hr before trials, which required the mouse to swim an alley way to escape from water and later to swim without escape but with a weight of 66.7 g/kg body weight attached to its tail for a prolonged period to avoid submersion through fatigue. For swimming speed to escape, the significant drug–coat-color interaction showed no systematic effects on the tendency of amphetamine to cause slower responding, and no effects whatsoever were detected for the swimming-to-exhaustion measure. While these findings and those from other tests not employing drugs have implications for major gene pleiotropism, they do not appear to bear on the coat-color–temperament hypothesis in the way that Keeler and Fromm (1965) claim their findings with foxes do. However, insufficient details of the derivation of the population of the amber coat-color mutant of the red foxes used, of the details of the various tranquilizing drugs administered, and, finally, of the standardization of the various observational procedures employed allow no evaluation of this work. These studies exemplify the truism that behavioral responses to drugs, typically quantitative in nature, are unlikely to be simply determined genetically by major genes, such as those for coat color, acting pleiotropically, and are much more likely to involve large numbers of genes, each minor in effect but acting additively (which includes subtractively) to produce the graded, quantitative phenotypes observed, as was stressed at the outset of this survey, and which require for their determination special analytical methods going beyond those available in major gene or mutation analysis. We shall return to this theme later.

Meanwhile, language difficulties can to some extent be held responsible for similar problems with a Russian psychopharmacogenetic study using dogs and the stimulant, caffeine (Isaeva and Krasuskii, 1961). The purpose here was doubtless the standard one in Pavlovian typological approaches (Gray, 1964) of using drugs to assist in classifying subjects according to type of nervous sytem. Thus dogs were judged as having a strong nervous system if they displayed no disruption of (unspecified) conditioned reflex activity by doses of 0.4 g of caffeine or more, and weak if disrupted by 0.3 or lower, but some genealogical relationships bearing on the inheritance of response to caffeine as determined in this way can be deduced. Ginsburg *et al.* (1976) briefly report variations following medication with amphetamine in the hyperkinesis displayed by hybrids between beagle dogs on the one hand and either coyotes or Telomian dogs on the other. In the latter cross amphetamine had a generally ameliorative effect, as opposed to barbiturates, which did not, whereas in the beagle–coyote cross it had no effect. Confirmation of the effect of amphetamine on the beagle–Telomian cross comes from Lucas and Scott (1977) who carried matters further with a reciprocal cross. Preliminary data suggest a maternal effect in that puppies showing increased restraint under the effects of amphetamine after inhibitory training are more numerous among a litter having a Telomian mother and a beagle father than the reciprocal cross in which the parental breeds were reversed.

Morrison and Stephenson (1973) used two groups of rats (Lister and a Lister/Sprague-Dawley cross) in an extensive study of the effects of amphetamine (and of nicotine) on various operant behavior schedules, but the numbers involved were probably too small to establish drug–strain interaction effects even if the data had been evaluated from this point of view, which they were not. Beckwith *et al.* (1974) contrasted Long-Evans hooded rats with albinos in a study of the effects of four dose levels of *d*-amphetamine on various aspects of learning and retention of a brightness discrimination. While strain differences were detected—the hooded rats with their pigmented irises being predictably better than the albinos with their transparent ones (lacking shielding melanin pigment)—drug–strain interactions were not detected.

Mention may most conveniently be made here of work by Lapin (1975) on apomorphine, a probable dopaminergic, on five different strains, three of them the same strains as in his previous work discussed above (BALB, C57BL, C57BR) augmented by C3H/A and an inbred Swiss strain, SHR. Behavioral measures were limited to ambulation and rearing, which were observed for 2 min in a cage 30 min after intraperitoneal injection of apomorphine in doses of 5, 10, 20, and 50 mg/kg. Clear drug–strain interaction was observed in both measures, which may be characterized by the statement that effects were generally inhibitory, especially at the highest dose level, except for the C57BL/6J mice, which showed stimulation of locomotion and to some extent of rearing at the lower doses. The distinctiveness of this strain from others is once again evident.

As part of a program of research concerned with the factors mediating the U-shaped function found in the retention of two-way escape–avoidance behavior based on shock, Barrett *et al.* (1973) also used Sprague–Dawley rats in a study that contrasted them with subjects from the Fischer strain with respect to their response to 2.0 mg/kg of *d*-amphetamine or 1.2 mg/kg of scopolamine and, later, to both together. In each case, the drugs were injected intraperitoneally 30 min before 25 daily trials in a discriminated Y-maze, in which rats were required to run to an illuminated rather than to a dark arm within 10 sec in order to avoid foot shock. It was found that the drug–strain interaction took the form of an increase in correct avoidance performance by the Sprague–Dawley rats, especially under the influence of the drugs in combination, as compared with the Fischers, who performed well under all conditions. This finding is interpreted as supporting the view that a specific learning deficit due to response to shock may be overcome pharmacologically, but does not add to our understanding of the genetic mechanisms involved therein.

Anisman and his group's extensive studies in this area have been concerned largely with the same two drugs, amphetamine and scopolamine, and three strains of mice, C57BL/6J, DBA/2J, and A/J. To this work they bring a degree of sophistication in the specification and testing of hypothetical drug mechanism hitherto little encountered in this review. But it must be remembered that causal explanation in terms of brain biochemistry does not solve the problems of genetic mechanisms: "Level of a particular neurotransmitter," for example, is a phenotype like any other and is itself amenable to genetic analysis by appropriate methods already touched on here, including, of course, selective breeding, as in Roderick's (1960) highly successful bidirectional selection for level of brain acetylcholinesterase in rats. But the group around Anisman have also made some progress in the direction of genetic as opposed to pharmacological analysis, as we shall see. Concerned especially with the role of biochemical changes and the part they play in maintaining the balance between different neurotransmitter systems, which may modulate behavior giving rise to the shock-induced U-shaped function referred to above, they sought to bring both drugs and strain differences as variables to bear on the problem. A series of investigations (see Anisman, 1975*d*, for review) included the establishment of strain differences in drug responses in a variety of behavioral phenotypes and the crossbreeding between the strains and the measurement of their progeny in the same situations and under similar drug influence. Thus Anisman (1975*a*) used the three mouse strains mentioned in a study of discriminated escape–avoidance conditioning in a Y-shaped apparatus similar to that used by Barrett *et al.* (1973). It required the subject to learn that of the two escape routes from shock thus presented, the illuminated one was correct, and hence safe from further shock, and not the dark one. A range of doses of 1.0, 2.0, or 3.0 mg/kg of scopolamine hydrobromide or the same doses of *d*-amphetamine sulfate was injected intraperitoneally 10 min before the commencement of 60 training trials and showed that the drug–strain interaction detected took the form of a failure of amphetamine to improve the performance of the C57BL mice, as it did that of the other two strains, and of scopolamine to do more than improve the A/J strain only. Neither drug affected the discrimination score on the test, and it was the differential measures of incorrect and incomplete responding that it allows which showed the drug–strain interaction in the initiation of responding. To discover if this interesting finding could be generalized to the more usual form of two-way shuttle-box avoidance conditioning in which no discrimination procedure is additionally involved, Anisman (1976*b*) repeated the experiment using the same strains and one only of each of the doses—3.0 mg/kg amphetamine and 2.0 mg/kg scopolamine—and the same apparatus but blocking off one of the arms of the Y, thus creating a somewhat more conventional pattern of shuttle box. He also varied the location of the alley light, which served as the conditioned stimulus, so that mice were required either to run towards it, as in the previous experiment, or away from it. The results replicated rather precisely those found before for the running towards the light, except that the amphetamine-treated mice of the C57 strain were now significantly poorer than saline controls. Under the running away from the light condition, on the other hand, there was little difference between the strains, and drug responses were confined to the A/J strain, in which both facilitated performance as before, and to the DBA strain, whose performance was disrupted by scopolamine. The fact that the A strain is albino and hence has generally poorer vision than either of the other two pigmented strains, whose acuity might be affected by drug-induced pupillary effects, suggests that this variable may be important in determining these results. But Anisman argues cogently that the effect of stimulus variables generally cannot account for the drug–strain interactions observed, which must therefore be regarded as fairly robust.

In a test of inhibitory avoidance, so called to differentiate it from the more usual passive avoidance, and in which the animal was required to inhibit movement in an open field under pain of 0.3-mA foot shock, it was found (Anisman, 1975*a*) that the C57BL strain was immune to the disruption that the single dose of amphetamine (3.0 mg/kg) caused in the required restraint of activity of the other two strains, while the scopolamine (2.0 mg/kg) affected all three in this way. Anisman and Kokkinidis (1975) extended the approach to exploratory and alternation behavior, as measured in a Y-maze, with no shock being involved in this case. It was shown that doses ranging from 1.0 to 10.0 mg/kg of the same two drugs did not differentially affect the amount of alternation between the strains, merely reducing it to around chance level, so that it became indifferent which arm of the maze a mouse entered after leaving another, instead of being a function of that which had previously been chosen. Indeed, some perseverative effects were observed with the highest doses of scopolamine. Overall locomotor activity as such was notable only for some dose-dependent effects of both drugs. This finding was confirmed in an apparently independent experiment (Anisman, 1975*b*, Experiment 3) using scopolamine only in a single dose level (10 mg/kg).

In further work Anisman and Kokkinidis (1975) attempted to affect the level of catecholamine and acetylcholine activity influenced by amphetamine by administering it in conjunction with enzyme inhibitors known to reduce norepinephrine or norepinephrine and dopamine. These were α-methyl-paratyrosine (α-MpT for short), an inhibitor of tyrosine hydroxylase, and *bis*-(4-methyl-*1*-homopiperazinylthiocarbonyl) disulfide (FLA-63), an inhibitor of dopamine-β-hydroxylase. They were injected (i.p.) in single doses of 200 mg/kg and 40 mg/kg, respectively, alone or in combination with *d*-amphetamine (10 mg/kg), 3 hr 25 min and 25 min, respectively, before testing, and the effects on alternation and activity in the Y-maze were observed as before. The results showed that neither of the enzyme inhibitors alone affected alternation; the effect of amphetamine in reducing alternation without inducing any strain-dependent effects was confirmed. Once again locomotor activity revealed interaction, this time a drug–strain one in that the significant reduction of the amphetamine-induced locomotor excitement by both α-MpT and FLA-63 was not seen in the DBA strain, whereas both the A/J and C57BL mice displayed the antagonistic effects in varying degrees. The enzyme inhibitors separately each reduced activity significantly only in the DBA mice; simple drug–strain interactions which nevertheless indicated that their ineffectiveness in antagonizing amphetamine in this strain cannot have been due to its insusceptibility to their effect. However, there was no such strain interaction in a study (Anisman and Cygan, 1975) that used only FLA-63, though in combination with amphetamine (same doses, etc., as before) the antagonism was largely ineffective in the A as well as in the DBA strain as previously noted. But the measure employed was now activity, this time as observed in an open-field test with a grid floor, together with the additional phenotype of response to shock administered after 10 min of exploration had been permitted, so that the results may not be strictly comparable. As the authors state, "The source for this interaction is unclear. On the one hand it may simply represent differential rates of drug metabolism, while on the other hand it may suggest that the involvement of dopamine and norepinephrine in modulating amphetamine effects differ across strains" (Anisman and Cygan, 1975, pp. 838–839).

Further work by Anisman *et al.* (1975) also employed the activity response to foot shock, and the same extended dose range as before was used except for one of the three experiments, in which the sizes were 10.0 mg/kg of amphetamine and 1.0 of scopolamine, with the same route of administration and dose interval as in the group's previous work. Amphetamine enhanced activity in all strains, especially after shock, and to some extent as an increasing function of the number of shocks, whereas scopolamine had little or no effect. Since the strains differ with respect to their undrugged behavioral response to shock, the size of drug-induced effects can be seen to vary. Again this finding was confirmed (Anisman, 1975*b*, Experiment 2) separately, using scopolamine only, but in two (1.0 and 10.0 mg/kg) doses. It was on this (essential) basis that a cross-breeding program for these same phenotypes was attempted (Anisman, 1976*a*), and it is to a consideration of this work, which is also summarized in Table X, that we must now turn.

Chapter 6

Crossbreeding: Diallel Cross

The diallel method used by Anisman (1976*a*) involves crossing each strain with every other reciprocally so that, as in this case, the use of three parental strains generates a 3 × 3 diallel table of family means in which the reciprocal crosses, by which prenatal maternal effects can be detected (see Section 9.1), are distributed symmetrically around the leading diagonal formed by the parental strains. Thus there are three F_1s and their reciprocals, a total of six families, which together with the three parental strains generate the ninefold table, and allow the consequent multiple comparisons.

Procedures akin to those described above (Anisman *et al.*, 1975) were applied to the 270 subjects of both sexes bred for the diallel cross, who were exposed to the open field before and after shock, under either control (saline) conditions or 1.0 mg/kg scopolamine or 10.0 mg/kg amphetamine. The data were analyzed first in terms of the parental strains, the results, broadly speaking, supporting the findings of the previous investigation restricted to this class of subjects only. The crosses were analyzed separately and the "mode of inheritance" classified according to the several relationships of the F_1s to their respective parental strains. This approach generates a picture of some complexity in which suggestions of maternal effects appear in some crosses under one of the three environments in which they were tested (saline, amphetamine, or scopolamine) and not in others, and in which dominance relationships are inferred from F_1 resemblances to parental-strain values. Clearly, significant drug–strain interactions are present, but the conclusion that different genetic mechanisms contribute to the phenotypic changes observed, though highly plausible, is not unequivocally supported by the analyses presented.

A further report (Anisman, 1975*c*) deals with three other phenotypes in the diallel cross. These were the two-way avoidance conditioning referred to above, together with one-way conditioning in the same apparatus, a circular one in which the mouse progressed from one segment to the next in each of the 50 trials given instead of being required to shuttle back and forth between two segments only, and finally the test of inhibitory avoidance in the open-field apparatus (Anisman, 1975*a*) in which, as noted above, the shock was given not after 10 min but whenever a crossing from one square to another, marked on the floor, was made. The number of shocks received—an inverse measure of the extent of the inhibitory learning—was one of the measures used, the other being latency to the *second* shock. Three separate experiments, each involving 90 mice of both sexes, were reported, and the dosage used varied from that in the previous diallel experiment reported (Anisman, 1976*a*) and described above, which was presumably an independent experiment also, otherwise potentially severe problems relating to previous drug experience and order effects of testing might have been expected. The scopolamine dosage was larger (2.0 mg/kg) and the amphetamine dose smaller (3.0 mg/kg), each being contrasted with a similar saline control.

Results were again presented in terms of strains and their several F_1 crosses in each of the three separate drug environments. Once again clear drug–strain interactions were detected, together with suggestions of maternal effects. Some degree of hybrid vigor was demonstrated, but little was attempted by way of genetic interpretation of the complexities shown in the differences in the way performance on the various tasks was affected by drugs. This is not surprising in view of the absence of any overall analysis by which the effects of environmental effects, such as the drug treatments, maternal influences, and genetic effects, generated by the strain and their hybrids, could be evaluated against each other.

These investigations are nevertheless important in that they are among the first reported to apply the diallel crossbreeding method to the genetics of drug responsivity in situations in which the possibility exists of assessing genotype–environment interaction. But the diallel cross method as a breeding design as used in this study must be sharply distinguished from the diallel analysis for which this design has been extensively employed in biometrical genetics (Mather and Jinks, 1971) for the analysis of the genetic structure of quantitative traits, and to some extent in psychogenetics (e.g., Broadhurst, 1960; Henderson, 1968). The analyses presented by Anisman do not exploit its potentialities. The successive pairwise comparison of parental strains and of reciprocal F_1s, first under placebo conditions and then under the standard single doses mentioned above, is a piecemeal approach that destroys the undoubted power of a method already shown to be capable of extension for behavioral work to the multivariate case with the incorporation of treatment variables (Fulker *et al.*, 1972), so that additional diallel tables can be generated for each new treatment condition, such as the drugs here used. Classification by "mode of inheritance"—itself a deservedly obsolete term in genetics—based on the mere phenotypic resemblance of filial crosses to their appropriate parental values is an uncertain procedure for several reasons, which to explore fully would take us too far from our present themes. But it may be briefly said that such resemblance, when many genes are involved (as is almost certainly the case here), does not give information about their dominance relationships, and this fact is recognized by the use of a special term, "potence," to describe this apparent dominance, which may be merely phenotypic. Much less is the heterosis reported in several of the crosses, which out-perform both parental strains, attributable to overdominance in any simple way. The reason in both cases is that the genes, increasers and decreasers, dominants and recessives, contributing to the level of the phenotypic expression observed in the offspring are likely to be unequally distributed among the various parental strains used, as a result of the inbreeding process by which they were established, so that without investigating the genetic architecture involved—at the very least to the extent of partitioning and assessing the additive and dominance genetic contributions to the phenotype—we cannot use parental and F_1 phenotypic resemblances to establish the existence of genetic dominance. And without establishing the extent, and the nature, of dominance—that is, whether it be directional and tending to push the phenotype to one extreme or ambidirectional and tending to stabilize the phenotype at an intermediate value—we cannot lend any experimental backing to speculations about the adaptive and possibly evolutionary significance of changes in behavior or of neurochemistry (Anisman, 1975*d*; Wilcock and Fulker, 1973), which is perhaps one of the most interesting and important features that the powerful biometrical methodology provides (Broadhurst, 1968; Broadhurst and Jinks, 1974). Finally, in none of this extensive work, though both sexes appear to have been used as subjects throughout, are sex differences reported. It is not clear whether or not the data were analyzed in such a way as to permit their appearance and if so whether none were shown to exist. This important point deserves further attention, since the breeding design adopted allows the possibilities of sex linkage and sex limitation of action to be studied.

In view of the caveats expressed in this somewhat lengthy aside, the findings of these pioneer attempts at crossbreeding for an essentially pharmacological phenotype will not be reviewed in further detail. These valuable data might nevertheless be amenable to biometrical analyses that could reveal subtleties doubtless inherent in the genetical architecture of responses to the drugs used.

Chapter 7

Strain Differences II: Nicotine, Anxiolytics, Convulsants, and Amnesics

The investigations of Anisman, summarized in Table X, have brought us a long way from the study of simple strain differences in response to amphetamine (and scopolamine) in rodents, but it is to such that we must now return with respect to agents of this kind. Oliverio *et al.* (1966) reported data on a differential effect of a 2.7 mg/kg dose of scopolamine on avoidance conditioning depending on strain: DBA mice showed a tenfold increase in avoidance responses, whereas merely a threefold increase was found for C3H/He subjects. But the interactive effect depended on original performance level: Well trained mice of both strains showed, by contrast, a similar (and considerable) decrement.

Van Abeelen and Strijbosch (1969; see also van Abeelen, 1974) studied two of the inbred mouse strains later used by Anisman, the C57BL/6 and the DBA/2, and an F_1 cross between them, for various aspects of their exploratory behavior in a novel situation (a large, relatively empty cage) in which they differ, the C57 generally being the more active. A range of doses was used in each case, 1.25–10.0 mg/kg for scopolamine and 18.75–150.0 μg/kg for physostigmine. No drug–strain interaction was observed with the second drug, but with scopolamine a decrease was found in the C57's responses and an increase in the DBA's responses. No attempt at genetic analysis based on parent–hybrid differences was attempted. Bovet and Oliverio (1973, also in Oliverio, 1974*b* and Oliverio and Bovet, 1975) cite data that replicate the C57 × DBA cross under the effects of scopolamine (2.5 and 5.0 mg/kg) and physostigmine (0.15 and 0.30 mg/kg), the former within the range of dosages used by van Abeelen and Strijbosch, and the latter almost so, but using a measure of activity derived from crossings in a tilt box. Both agents caused changes in activity over control levels, but the only marked increase (about 20%) was detected in DBA animals, and the F_1 cross under both doses of scopolamine suggested potence, that is, phenotypic dominance for that inbred strain's response to this drug. Substituting in a similar cross with C57BL a different inbred mouse strain, the SEC/1ReJ, gave a not dissimilar pattern of results, though the increase now reached over 100% in the SEC's and the F_1's response to the larger dose of scopolamine. Physostigmine, on the other hand, generally depressed activity for all strains and crosses, as did scopolamine for the C57's, findings that overall support those of van Abeelen and Strijbosch (1969). Extending this approach to amphetamine yielded data of some interest in that here again it was the C57 mice that showed reduced activity in response to both of the doses used (0.5 and 1.0 mg/kg), whereas the other two strains involved in the F_1 crosses, the DBA and the SEC, both showed modest increases. But the F_1 values themselves differed, resembling the C57 more in the case of the first cross but the SEC in the case of the latter. No analyses, even of phenotypic values, resulting in significance levels were presented, so that the evidence for the conclusions that ". . . cholinergic and adrenergic mechanisms seem to be regulated by two different genetic factors" (Bovet and Oliverio, 1973, p. 25) must remain in doubt for the moment. It should also be noted that the *decrease* in activity after amphetamine in the C57BL/6J mice is an unusual finding, not replicated in other work reported by this group (Oliverio *et al.*, 1973a). Dosages including those previously used (0.5 and 1.0 mg/kg), and extending to 2.0 mg/kg, showed clear dose-dependent increases, though in a slightly different substrain, the C57BL/6By (see also Chapter 8).

In order to determine whether the postulated cholinergic mechanism facilitating exploration is central or peripheral, van Abeelen *et al.* (1971) also employed quaternary congeners of the two drugs previously used, scopolamine methylbromide and neostigmine bromide, since they both pass the blood–brain barrier only poorly. Intravenous injections of 5.2 mg/kg and 58.4 μg/kg, respectively, were given 30 min prior to exposure to the exploratory test. The findings successfully replicated those of the previous experiment with respect to the central acting drugs: The peripheral ones had no effect in general, thus supporting the basic proposition of central cholinergic facilitation. To confirm if its location might be central as conjectured, van Abeelen *et al.* (1972) injected the latter drugs directly into the hippocampus, thus bypassing the blood–brain barrier, in the way previously noted (Chapter 4) for methylscopolamine only. Two dose levels were used, and the same exploratory situation as before, though with a modified but still empty food hopper. Neostigmine now had the same effects as did physostigmine in that it uniformly depressed activity, irrespective of strain, whereas methylscopolamine now mimicked scopolamine in increasing DBA activity and decreasing that of the C57BL mice, at least in the lower dose of 7.8 µg per mouse. Work specifically oriented toward the exploration of the genetical determinants of the behavioral phenotypes manipulated by this elegant but difficult technique has been furthered by use of the two selected strains derived by van Abeelen (1970) from a cross between the C57BL and the DBA and already described (Chapter 4).

Anisman and Cygan (1975) also employed the same technique as van Abeelen in order to see whether central rather than peripheral mechanisms mediate the modification by scopolamine and amphetamine of the effects on activity in the open-field test caused by foot shock. They used the procedure described in Section 5.2 and the three strains favored by Anisman's group, the A/J, DBA/2J, and C57BL/6J strains. Intraperitoneal injections of scopolamine hydrobromide (dosages of 1.0, 5.0, and 10.0 mg/kg) or d-amphetamine sulfate (same doses) were matched by groups of mice receiving scopolamine methylsulfate (0.9, 4.5, and 9.0 mg/kg) or p-hydroxyamphetamine hydrobromide (0.63, 3.15, and 6.30 mg/kg), respectively. Both of the peripherally acting agents were without effect on activity scores both prior to and in response to foot shock, thus confirming the central action of the other two. Scopolamine and amphetamine gave results that broadly confirmed previously reported findings, and so strengthened the evidence for their differential strain-limited effects. Further support comes from an interesting developmental study (Remington and Anisman, 1976) in which the effects of scopolamine (0.5 and 1.0 mg/kg) and amphetamine (same two dosages plus 5.0 mg/kg) were observed on the open-field unshocked activity not of adults of the three strains, but of juveniles of 14, 21, and 28 days. Activity was automatically recorded for 10 min, beginning 10 min after the drug treatment. The outcomes were quite clear: Scopolamine gave a significant increase in activity which developed with age but the time of onset was strain dependent in that at age 14 days none showed it; at age 21 days the DBA was the only strain to show it significantly whereas at 28 days all did. In contrast, amphetamine occasioned an increase that, though only in the hightest dose (5.0 mg/kg), was evidenced significantly at 14 days in all except the DBA mice, but which was seen in all strains thereafter. These interactions of the strain-limited drug responses with age were related by the authors to differential maturation of the biochemical systems underlying the actions of scopolamine as an anticholinergic drug and d-amphetamine as a catecholamine stimulant.

Cazala's work (1976) breaks new ground in two ways: First, he used a phenotype not hitherto encountered in this monograph, the intensity of intracranial self-stimulation, and second, he compared the *d*- and *l*-isomers of amphetamine. After stereotaxic implantation of bipolar electrodes into the dorsal or the ventral lateral hypothalamus of male mice of three strains (C57BL/6, DBA/2, and BALB/c), all of the Orl substrains, they were tested in cages provided with two levers. One merely recorded bar-pressing activity as such, the other was connected to devices that delivered low intensities of electric current to the animal's brain, enabling the self-stimulation threshold intensity to be measured, after which an increased current was used to maintain bar-pressing behavior. Doses of both isomers of amphetamine were the same for all strains, starting at 0.25 mg/kg injected intraperitoneally 20 min after the beginning of each 2-hr test session, with doses increasing by doubling the initial value until motor disturbance was observed. The strains were differentially sensitive in this respect, the C57 mice tolerating 8.0 mg/kg, the DBA mice 2.0 mg/kg, and the BALB mice only 1.0 mg/kg. The effect of the drug varied with isomer, the *l*-isomer being less potent in its facilitatory effects and more potent in its depressing effects on self-stimulation counts, as well as with electrode positioning—the dorsal generally showing the more striking efforts than the ventral position, the placements being checked histologically. In addition there was an interaction with strain, which, broadly speaking, followed the strain sensitivities mentioned above in that the largest effects were seen in the C57 mice and were less marked in the DBA and BALB strains.

Lapin (1974) also briefly reports on experiments suggestive of interaction with strain in response to cholinergic drugs, and the effect of physostigmine on exploratory behavior in a novel situation was also observed by Morrison and Lee (1968) in a comparative study employing three strains of rats, Sprague–Dawley, Lister, and Wistar, as subjects. Its action was contrasted with that of nicotine on the grounds that if nicotine's central action can be postulated as similar to that of physostigmine as a cholinergic drug (cholinesterase inhibitor), then the variations induced by the two drugs in the behavioral phenotypes observed should be similar. In general, this expectation was borne out, the more active Lister rats being more depressed by the subcutaneous dose of 0.4 mg/kg of nicotine used than either of the other strains, but there was considerable within-strain variability in this long-term (27 weeks) experiment and the results for physostigmine were less clear cut. Nevertheless, a degree of drug–strain interaction can be accepted as having been demonstrated.

7. 1. Nicotine

In further work using nicotine, Silverman (1971) studied the effects on social behavior among rats of a minimal or "smoking" dose of nicotine (25 μg/kg), using two strains, Wistar-derived albinos and an unspecified black-hooded strain. No interaction was detected, the response to the drug being reported as very similar in the two strains. Such was not the case in an extensive study of ten different mouse strains by Bovet *et al.* (1966), nine of them being inbreds and all included among those so far mentioned in this book. The behavior examined was acquisition and performance of two-way escape–avoidance conditioning extending over five days of 100 trials each, and 0.5 mg/kg of nicotine sulfate was given intraperitoneally 15 min before each session lasting at least 50 min. The data indicate that overall performance was affected by the drug in a way that reflected a marked drug–strain interaction. There was a definite tendency for nicotine to improve acquisition and performance in low-avoiding strains, which scored successful responses on one third or fewer of the trials and this group of six included BALB/c and a genetically heterogeneous Swiss strain—but among the four high-scoring strains (one third or more avoidances) two patterns emerged. Typical were the C57BL/10, which were significantly poorer under the drug, the DBA/2J alone differing with an increase in its already high (one half successful) performances. It is noted that two sets of three each of the strains are closely related in their derivation from foundation stocks yet differ in the level of their undrugged performance and, in one of the groups, also in the direction of their response to nicotine. The effects of arecoline are briefly reported by Bovet *et al.* (1969) as not paralleling the effects of nicotine on two of the strains, the DBA/2J and the BALB/c, in that none of a series of doses ranging from 0.5 to 4.0 mg/kg had any facilitatory effect.

Four of the inbred strains of mice were also used by Bovet-Nitti (1969) to assess the effects of nicotine on another task, that of acquiring a visual discrimination of an avoidance kind in which the mouse had to choose the correctly designated door out of five, four being marked with the same incorrect symbol, in order to escape shock. Nicotine in the same dosage and administration procedure as before improved performance significantly, for one or another of the two sets of symbols used, in all strains except the BALB/c, but the patterning of this drug–strain interaction was, as might be expected, not the same for this behavioral phenotype as for the shuttle-box conditioning previously studied. For example, the A/J strain, which previously showed a decrement, was improved by nicotine with respect to visual discrimination. Nevertheless, as before, it was the high-scoring strain, in this case BALB/c, whose performance was disrupted. Possible major gene influence can be detected in these results in that the C3H/He mice (some lines of which carry the gene for retinal degeneration, a mutation of obvious importance in a visual task), while performing well under massed practice (intertrial time interval not stated), showed a failure of performance when the number of successive daily trials was reduced from ten to three. Position habits, though claimed to be absent in mice, could be of greater assistance to subjects with impaired vision given a longer practice period, especially if the correct door was not varied between trials, but merely between sessions. Neither is this important procedural point stated in her paper on the same technique in rats (1966), discussed earlier (Chapter 4).

Castellano (1976) used the DBA/2J and C57BL/6J strains to study the effects of nicotine on swimming behavior toward or away from a light. Automatic Y-shaped water mazes required the mouse to swim from one arm to the choice point where the presence of a light in one of the other arms could be detected. It indicated the presence or absence of an escape platform beneath it, depending on whether light or dark was the cue for the arm designated correct. The effects of pretrial injections of 0.25, 0.5, and 1.0 mg/kg of nicotine tartrate (route unspecified) 30 min beforehand on the acquisition of both types of learning, and of immediate posttrial injections of 0.5 mg/kg on learning the dark-correct requirement, were presented in a series of graphs and evaluated by multiple comparisons for significant differences between groups. A more efficient statistical analysis might render more secure the conclusion that there exists a drug–strain interaction in the pretrial treatments in the dark-correct mode, though not in the light-correct, in that learning in it is impaired in the DBA mice and enhanced in the C57 mice. The effect was most marked at the intermediate dose, the 0.25 mg/kg dose having uniformly nonsignificant effects and the 1.0 mg/kg dose uniformly inhibitory ones, as compared with saline injections in all cases. The effects of this 0.5 mg/kg dose were precisely comparable when given immediately after each session of five trials at 1-min intervals, though a delay of 2 hr before injection failed to have any significant effect on either strain. The effect of nicotine on mice trained to a criterion of 100% correct choices was not fully reported, so that it was not possible to ascertain the existence or otherwise of a drug–strain interaction for this phenotype.

Nicotine was used by Hatchell and Collins (1977) in a study in which the exploratory activity of two sublines of DBA and C57BL mice, the /2Ibg and the /6Ibg strains, respectively, was observed 5 min after 1 mg/kg nicotine. Sex differences in both behavior and concentrations in the liver and brain were especially prominent, whereas if the nicotine was injected after 2, 4, or 7 days of pretreatment with thrice daily doses, strain differences were also revealed as important, with DBA males showing the least development of tolerance and C57BL males the most to the decrease in exploration observed.

These findings may be compared with those of Rosecrans and Schechter (1972) with rats. They found the Sprague–Dawley and Fischer strains differed in measures of general activity immediately after a subcutaneous injection of 400 μg/kg of nicotine, the Fischers showing the greater increases over water-injected controls. But in both strains the increases were significant among females only, which was also true of measures of the accumulation of the drug in various brain tissues. Table XI summarizes the experimentation concerned with nicotine.

This concludes our survey of broadly stimulant drugs as modulated in their effects by genetic variables. It cannot be claimed that generalizations spring readily to mind, but there is considerable evidence of the existence of the raw material for genetic analyses in the strain differences detected and some, albeit as yet faltering but nonetheless definite, steps towards a proper genetic analysis of genotype–environment interaction by appropriate crossing methods, as exemplified by the work of Anisman.

7.2. Anxiolytics and Other Agents

Other classes of pharmacological agents do not rival those we have previously considered with respect to the volume of work published on them using inbred strains. But among the anxiolytics, chlorpromazine has been widely used, for example in a relatively early study of strain differences in drug responsivity in mice. Huff (1962) briefly reported an important study (apparently employing the diallel cross method), in which four inbred strains, including the C57BL/6J and the DBA/2J and all possible filial crosses, were tested for 3 min 20 sec in an automatically recorded activity apparatus 1 hr after a range of four doses, 0.5 mg/kg being the smallest and 4.0 mg/kg the largest. The summary tantalizingly reports that "Results show differential sensitivity of genotypes superimposed on a general depressant effect," but the further details given do little to support the assertion that a simple genetic mechanism might be responsible for the drug responses observed and no further report has subsequently come to hand.

Bourgault *et al.* (1963) contrasted C57BL/6 mice with another inbred but albino strain called SC-I in a series of tests that included the measurement of behavioral phenotypes relating to activity as observed in various devices, along with escape latency to periodic shock in one of them. The activity measures all showed that the black strain, while more active than the SC-I in saline control conditions, was more responsive to intraperitoneal doses of a range of 2.0 to 10.0 mg/kg of chlorpromazine in terms of reduction in activity and escape. Meier *et al.* (1963), as already noted (Section 5.2), used chlorpromazine as part of their study of four mouse strains and found that only among the DBA mice did a single dose of 1.0 mg/kg do more than compensate for the saline-injection-induced depression of activity by showing an increase, sustained over the 30-min test, and significantly different from that of the other three strains. A dose of 0.95 mg/kg was

TABLE XI

Psychopharmacogenetic Experiments with Nicotine, Anxiolytics, and Other Agents

Reference	Species (and strain)	Drug	Measure	Outcome	Remarks
Silverman (1971)	Rats, Wistar albino and black hooded	Nicotine	Social behavior	No drug–strain interaction	
Bovet et al. (1966)	Mice, 10 different strains	Nicotine sulfate	Two-way escape conditioning	Drug–strain interaction. Drug improved conditioning of low-avoidance strains	Varying patterns of response, consistent for certain strains. Arecoline effects different (Bovet et al., 1969)
Bovet-Nitti (1969)	Mice, 4 strains	Nicotine	Visual discrimination	Drug–strain interaction. Nicotine improved performance of all but BALB/c	Patterning of interaction different again
Castellano (1976)	Mice, DBA/2J, C57BL/6J	Nicotine tartrate	Swimming to or from light	Drug–strain interaction reported. C57 learn better than DBA under nicotine	Statistical analysis?
Hatchell and Collins (1977)	Mice, DBA/2Ibg, C57BL/6Ibg	Nicotine bitartrate	Exploratory activity (also bioassay)	Sex differences and drug–strain interaction. C57BL develop tolerance >DBA (males)	Compare findings with rats (Rosecrans and Schechter, 1972)
Huff (1962)	Mice, 4 strains and all F₁ crosses	Chlorpromazine	Activity	"Differential sensitivity of genotypes. . . general depressant effect"	
Bourgault et al. (1963)	Mice, C57BL/6, SC-I	Chlorpromazine	Activity and escape latency	C57BL more active in control conditions, more susceptible to drug reduction of activity	
Meier et al. (1963)	Mice, 4 strains	Chlorpromazine	Activity	Only DBA increased	
van Abeelen (1966)	Mice, 6 strains	Chlorpromazine	Fur shaking	Drug effect but no drug–strain interaction	
Fuller (1966)	Mice, 3 strains, including C57BL	Chlorpromazine	Avoidance response Activity of yoked controls	Drug–strain interaction No interaction	

Reference	Animal/strain	Drug	Measure	Results	Comments
Fuller (1970*b*)	Mice, 4 strains	Chlorpromazine Chlordiazepoxide	Passive avoidance Active (Sidman) avoidance	No drug-strain interaction Drug-strain-dose interaction	
Sansone and Messeri (1974)	Mice, BALB/c, SEC/1Re	Chlorpromazine, chlordiazepoxide	Active (two-way) avoidance	Drug-strain interaction suggested	No assessment of drug-strain interaction possible
Fuller and Clark (1966)	Dogs	Chlorpromazine	Fear and socialization	No interaction	
Scott (1974)	Dogs, beagles, Telomians, and F_1 cross	Imipramine	Distress vocalization	Potence (phenotypic dominance) for non-response to drug	Order effects?
Lapin (1967)	Mice, C57BL, C57BR, and BALB	Imipramine Atropine Benactyzine	Rearing	No interaction C57BL increased BALB increased	
Lapin (1974)	Mice, C57BL, C57BR, and BALB	Imipramine	Locomotion Aggression	C strains increased but not BALB	
Lush (1975*a*)	Mice, 7 strains	Mescaline hemisulfate	Open-field defecation	Defecation reduced	
Lush (1975*b*)	Mice, 7 strains	Hexobarbitone	Sleep time	Results correlated with mescaline effect above	
Stasik and Kidwell (1969)	Mice, 4 strains and reciprocal crosses	LSD-25 tartrate	T-maze learning	Genotype-environment interaction (LSD depression interacts with additive genetic determination). Heterosis demonstrated	Brief report but complete diallel cross
Rambert *et al.* (1976)	Mice, 6 strains, including 2 CHs	Meprobamate Diazepam, oxazepam	Activity and shock	No strain difference Drug-strain interaction	
Tilson *et al.* (1976)	Rats, Fischer, Sprague-Dawley	LSD	Response rate on FI schedule Shock avoidance	Stimulated response Depressed	Barrett *et al.* (1973) findings confirmed
		Amphetamine		Drug-strain interaction Few strain differences	

found by van Abeelen (1966) to differentiate drugged mice from saline controls with respect to the incidence of fur shaking, but there was little evidence that the effect varied over the six strains studied.

In a careful investigation of the effects of chlorpromazine on performance of active (shuttle) avoidance in a Sidman avoidance situation, Fuller (1966) found that mice of three strains, including the C57BL but not the DBA, responded differentially to the same range of doses as used earlier by Huff (1962)—see above—when avoidance measures of experimental animals were considered, but not when the activity of the randomly shocked yoked control subjects was in question. In a further study using both chlorpromazine and chlordiazepoxide, Fuller (1970*b*) failed to find any differential effects of strain as such among four strains of mice in a passive-avoidance task. Similarly, for the active (Sidman) avoidance, only the interaction of the linear regression of doses of chlordiazepoxide with strains reached significance, the data suggesting that the increasing progression of doses of this drug (5.0, 10.0, and 20.0 mg/kg) tended to depress activity in the high-scoring strains such as the DBA/2J and RF/J while enhancing it in the low, C57BL/J strain.

Sansone and Messeri's study (1974) used the same two drugs to investigate the differences between the active-avoidance (two-way) conditioning of two other strains which had been shown to differ, the BALB/c and the SEC/1Re strains. Dose–response curves were established for both drugs, with the BALB mice being uniformly more sensitive than the SEC, which suggested a definite drug–strain interaction.

Fuller and Clark (1966) have also used chlorpromazine in attempts to modify behavioral phenotypes in another animal, the dog, the genetic variable here being breed, which may be viewed as the outcome of genetic selection by dog breeders for characteristics, including behavioral ones, the details of which were not recorded and were, in some cases, procedures of considerable antiquity (Scott and Fuller, 1965). However, once again no interaction between drug and breed was detected in a careful study of the effects of isolation during early life on measures of fear and socialization at 20 weeks of age. Dosages of 10–12 mg/kg were given 1 hr before behavioral testing. Scott (1974) used the antidepressant, imipramine, to study distress vocalization in, among others, beagles and Telomians, for which an F_1 cross was also available. While the beagles showed some reduction in vocalization in response to 8.0 mg/kg, neither the Telomians nor the Telomian × beagle cross showed any, which suggests considerable potence (phenotypic dominance) for the nonresponsiveness displayed by the mother's breed.

Lapin (1974), again using the same three inbred strains of mice as previously cited (Section 5.2), the C57BL, C57BR, and BALB strains, showed that imipramine (25 mg/kg) increased aggression among the latter two, but not the first, having previously shown (Lapin, 1967) that a rearing test given 30 min after 14 mg/kg did not differentiate them. In contrast, it was only the C57BL mice that showed an increase in rearing, which reached significance after the same dose of atropine. Benactyzine, on the other hand, in the same dose showed the increase only among the BALB mice; the C57BR mice were not included in this comparison, however. Locomotory activity measures, recorded automatically, were also taken from these strains after treatment with the same drugs, but the data were not presented in such a way as to enable the assessment of the significance of possible drug–strain interactions, and in any case emphasis was less on the genetic determinants of drug response than on the suitability or otherwise of particular strains for drug assay. Similar considerations were evident in Rambert *et al.*'s study (1976) in which various substrains, six in number and including two CH strains, were given behavioral tests including spontaneous and shock-inhibited activity as well as electroconvulsive shock. Meprobamate did not differentiate the strains, but the benzodiazepines, diazepam and oxazepam, did, the CH-derived strains showing greater depression of activity than most of the other Swiss mouse strains.

An extensive survey of seven mouse strains, six inbred and one other, and their response to mescaline has been reported (Lush, 1975a) using defecation in the open-field situation as the dependent variable. Intraperitoneal injection of 35 mg/kg of mescaline hemisulfate appeared to reduce defecation, but in view of the questionable validity of this measure as an index of emotionality in the mouse (Bruell, 1969)—as opposed to the rat—together with the possibility that order effects may have affected the results, there being no tests of concurrently nondrugged controls, the implications of these findings are uncertain. However, the strong correlation reported (Lush, 1975b) between hexobarbitone sleep times in these same strains and the action of mescaline are noteworthy. Variation in subcellular morphology, especially the microsomal system, which may be involved in the metabolism of both drugs, is suspected. No comparison with Vesell's (1968) results using a related barbiturate (see Section 7.3) are possible because the ranges of mouse strains used have only one (C3H/He) in common.

The effect of another hallucinogen, LSD, also in comparison with another drug, this time amphetamine, was investigated by Tilson *et al.* (1976), who used two strains of rats, the Fischer albino and the Sprague–Dawley hooded strains. The measures employed were rate of responding to food reinforcement at fixed (60 sec) intervals (FI schedule) in a Skinner box and unsignaled shock avoidance, also based on a bar-pressing response. After baselines had been established—which showed that the Sprague–Dawley rats responded faster than the Fischers to the FI 60 schedule, but more slowly in the avoidance task, broadly confirming Barrett *et al.*'s (1973) findings for these two strains (see Section 5.2)—a range of doses of each drug was tested. Intraperitoneal injections of 0.10, 0.20, 0.50, and 1.00 mg/kg of *d*-LSD tartrate immediately before testing showed that FI responding was generally stimulated, significantly so for both strains at intermediate doses, whereas the major effect on avoidance was depressive, the Sprague–Dawleys being significantly more affected than the Fischers at the two highest doses used (0.40 and 0.80 mg/kg in this case). A rather clear drug–strain interaction was thus demonstrated. With *d*-amphetamine in doses ranging from 0.75 to 1.0 mg/kg, on the other hand, little was found by way of strain differences in the overall dose–response curves, which showed a stimulation of the FI responding at the lower doses, depression of it at the highest, and an overall stimulation of avoidance responding. The data suggest, however, a significantly greater increase in avoidance among the Fischer rats, in contrast with the previous finding.

Further work on the effect of LSD on learning a T-maze was investigated by Stasik and Kidwell (1969). They used four inbred mouse strains and their F_1 crosses, bred reciprocally in the complete diallel-cross design, which was replicated six times. Half of each sex among each of the 16 litters constituting it were injected with 0.4 mg/kg of LSD tartrate 2 min before commencing training in a T-maze in which the box, runway, and the arm of the T designated as incorrect were electrified. The criterion of learning was nine successive correct trials and appropriate arrangements were made for discarding nonlearners. Insofar as can be judged from the necessarily condensed description presented in their rather brief report, Stasik and Kidwell applied relatively sophisticated biometrical analyses of the various response measures recorded and the conclusion that a genotype–environment interaction, where the latter component was a drug response, had been demonstrated was based on evidence superior to any other currently available in the literature. The overall depression of learning occasioned by LSD clearly interacts with additive genetic determination, though differently according to which of the behavioral phenotypes is being analyzed, and there is some evidence of heterosis for most of the five measures reported. The analysis used excludes the determination of dominance variation, so that the direction of dominance with the important clues it provides to the evolution of the character investigated cannot be evaluated from this nevertheless interesting study.

This concludes the survey of strain differences in mice and dogs in response to anxiolytic and some other drugs, and the outcomes are also summarized in Table XI. Once again only the sketchiest outlines of drug–strain interactions can be determined save in isolated reports, of which Stasik and Kidwell's (1969) is clearly the most important.

7.3. Convulsants, Anticonvulsants, and Amnesics

While it is not intended in this book to review the genetics of audiogenic seizures as such and their biochemical basis in laboratory or other rodents, some examples may be noted of genotype–drug interactions involved in the determination of this response to intense sound stimulation of an unusual kind, outside the range of that which the species may normally be expected to encounter. Thus the effects of three convulsing agents, cardiazol, strychnine, and caffeine (in very large doses) are briefly reported by Busnel and Lehmann (1961) using mice from the same Swiss albino lines, some audiogenic seizure prone and others resistant, though it is not clear from the brief report if these subjects constitute different sublines and, if so, how they originated. Dose–response differences in seizure threshold congruent with expectation were found. In the opposite sense, the protective effects of chlorpromazine have been studied in two susceptible strains of mice by Plotnikoff (1960, 1963b) who contrasted the inbred DBA/1 with the inbred Swiss albino and found that while a relatively small dose of 4.8 mg/kg was effective in preventing seizures in 50% of the DBA animals, up to 160.0 mg/kg had no protective effect among the Swiss mice. Meprobamate had a similar differential effect, but reserpine was equally effective among both. But if a heterogeneous stock of Swiss mice was used (Plotnikoff, 1963b), it was found that chlorpromazine protected them too and data were presented that indicate the progressive diminution of this protection over some 13 generations as inbreeding by brother × sister mating progressed, concurrently, presumably with selection for seizure susceptibility. This interesting example of a genotype–environment interaction in the making, so to speak, does not appear to have been followed up and it may be because the inbred–noninbred distinction in seizure susceptibility is not especially secure, as one of the discussants of this paper asserted (Plotnikoff, 1963b, p. 444). Additional work on the escape or initial running component only of audiogenic seizure in the mouse using various drugs is reported (also in Plotnikoff, 1963a) without further interaction of their effects with the DBA and Swiss strains used.

In the extensive work of Schlesinger and his group on this topic, the strain difference between DBA and C57Bl mice has, on the other hand, proven to be quite robust. The former are a dilute strain, carrying the major coat-color gene, *d*, for which they are doubly recessive, whereas the latter have its normal expression. Schlesinger *et al.* (1968a; Schlesinger and Griek, 1970) confirmed that the DBA/2J strain are more susceptible to seizures and showed that reserpine sensitizes both this strain and the C57BL/6J strain used as the other parent, as well as the F_1 cross between them. Seizure susceptibility was enhanced, especially among the DBA mice, 2 hr after a dose of 1 mg/kg. These findings were extended to electrically induced seizures using the parental strains only (Schlesinger *et al.*, 1968*c*) and to chemically induced seizures occasioned by pentylenetetrazol. No especially clear-cut drug–strain interactions were detected: The two parental strains, broadly speaking, retained their respective status, with the F_1 intermediate. Tetrabenazine has also been used to increase susceptibility (Schlesinger *et al.*, 1968*a*; Schlesinger and Griek, 1970) with similar effect on audiogenic responses, but alpha-methyl tyrosine and *para*-chlorophenylalanine showed a somewhat different effect in that both the DBA and the hybrids were affected, whereas the C57 mice remained resistant. The effects of 5-hydroxytryptophan, intended to raise the levels of brain serotonin in contrast to the previous treatment shown, with the exception of alpha-methyl tyrosine, to lower them (Schlesinger and Griek, 1970), were also investigated in these strains using two of the methods of convulsing mice described. But only parental values were reported for the electrical stimuli, with the F_1 added for the chemical method. Again no differential departures from the undrugged phenotype were found, the treatment being generally protective. Direct intracranial injection of serotonin (and of norepinephrine), on the other hand, showed a protective effect against audiogenic seizures in both inbred strains, but not their cross (Schlesinger and Griek, 1970). A monoamine oxidase inhibitor, iproniazid, gave protection against seizures resulting from pentylenetetrazol, but it was the F_1 generation that again showed themselves unresponsive to amino-oxyacetic acid, which afforded protection against the convulsant. Both of the inbred strains, given the same dosage of 20.0 μg/g 7 hr before being challenged with 78.0 mg/kg of pentylenetetrazol, showed significant reduction in the number of animals convulsing (Schlesinger *et al.*, 1968*b*). Schlesinger and Griek (1970) did not comment on these interesting findings, which indicated that some differential responsivity in the filial cross may be a function of their (uniformly) heterozygous genotype. They provided a useful summary of their findings (1970, p. 249), but limited their discussion of the psychogenetic aspects of seizures as revealed by their extensive experiments to a consideration of the bearing they have on the hypothesis implicating the major gene difference in coat color provided by the dilute (*d*) locus as a determining factor. They judged that the weight of evidence points away from any direct connection between *d* and seizure susceptibility. Boggan and Seiden (1971) confirmed the reserpine enhancement of audiogenic seizure susceptibility in the DBA/2 strain referred to above and showed that it also applied to another subline, DBA/1. Both were also equally susceptible to the effects of a dose of 200 mg/kg of 3, 4-dihydroxyphenylalanine (L-dopa), which antagonized the effect.

Bovet and Oliverio (1973) cite data (see also Oliverio, 1974b) that confirm and extend the findings of Schlesinger's group to another mouse strain, SEC/1ReJ, by showing that such mice also have the lower thresholds to the same chemical and electrical convulsants as do the DBA/2J, but not the C57BL/6J strains. Crosses, between the C57 and the other two strains individually, gave dose–response curves to each treatment, which broadly resembled the C57, in the case of the cross with the DBA, and the SEC, in the case of the cross with that strain.

Chemically induced convulsions as such, that is, those unrelated to audiogenic seizure susceptibility, have also been shown to be strain dependent. In the investigations by Meier *et al.* (1963) and Bourgault *et al.* (1963) previously referred to (Sections 5.2 and 7.2, respectively), pentylenetetrazol was infused continuously until convulsion occurred in the first case and injected intraperitoneally (60.0 mg/kg) in the second. Latency measures showed little difference between the SC-I and C57BL/6 mice used by Bourgault *et al.* (1963), whereas the latter strain was the most resistant of the four used by Meier *et al.* (1963), with the BALB/c and the C3H/An mice being most sensitive in terms of latency to, and duration of, convulsions. Sedation (by pentobarbital, same dosage and route) showed a dissimilar pattern, with the DBA/2 mice being the most protected. Another barbiturate, phenobarbital sodium, in three doses ranging from 75.0 to 150.0 mg/kg, reversed the significant difference in activity measures between the two strains in Bourgault *et al.*'s experiment, while reserpine (1.25 and 2.5 mg/kg, intraperitoneally) reduced activity more in the low-scoring C57BL/6 mice, also found to be more persistently responsive to the drug's effect over five days. Davis (Davis and Webb, 1963, 1964; Davis and King, 1967) has explored the effects of the convulsant hexafluorodiethyl ether (flurothyl). A circadian rhythm in responsivity interacted only with the initial convulsive phenomena in one experiment, but in another clear-cut strain differences were detected, with DBA/2 mice being the least, and C57BL/6 and BALB/c mice being the most, resistant to convulsion among the six strains given flurothyl (Davis and King, 1967).

Reverting to the more behavioral topic of audiogenic seizures, from which we have strayed, Boggan *et al.* (1971) studied the acoustic priming effect (see Schlesinger and Sharpless, 1975, for review). This effect, by which mice can be sensitized to become seizure prone by early brief exposure to sound, was investigated to detect differences between strains and sensitivity to drugs. They used the C57BL/6 inbred strain and McClearn's HS, a genetically heterozygous stock derived originally from an eight-way cross of eight well-established strains. After determining the optimal parameters for the study of the priming effect, which differed in that the HS were most sensitive to priming at 18 days of age as opposed to the C57's 20 days, and to a test–retest interval of 2 as opposed to 8 days, Boggan and his colleagues used several agents on both strains. Unfortunately, only one, 5-hydroxytryptophan (150 mg/kg), was common to both and, as it uniformly produced decreased seizure response to the sound, no drug–strain interaction was detected. However, Maxson *et al.* (1975), part of the group of workers associated with Ginsburg, who has contributed so largely to the understanding of the genetic pathways governing seizure susceptibility in the mouse, have briefly reported that amino-oxyacetic acid prevents acoustic priming in the C57 strain, whereas it does not in the DBA strain. Again, cycloheximide—an inhibitor of protein synthesis in the brain and elsewhere—protects the former strain but not the latter against seizure induction procedure as such. Since Yanai and Ginsburg also briefly report (1973) that the essentially life-long forced ingestion of ethanol differentially increased the seizure susceptibility of the offspring of two inbred strains, the C57 blacks being more affected than the DBA, and Yanai *et al.* (1975) in yet another brief report indicate that cross-fostering procedures have shown that the effect is induced postnatally, the basis for further analysis of these interesting phenotypes is clearly being laid.

As with the rat, mouse strains have been used to investigate memory, pharmacologically. Krivanek and McGaugh (1968) also used pentylenetetrazol, this time in subconvulsive doses of 5, 10, or 20 mg/kg, administered to mice of the C57BL/6 and BALB/c strains immediately after each of seven daily trials run for a food reward in a Lashley III maze. The drug had a generally facilitative effect on learning, but the lowest dose was clearly the optimum for the C57 mice. A different, single mouse strain (Swiss-albino) or rats were used in the other work reported using this drug, and it was left to Buckholtz (1974) to pursue this clear drug–strain interaction. But using DBA/2J mice with which to compare the C57BL/6J and a different learning task (20 trials daily of escape–avoidance conditioning in a shuttle box) he found no comparable interaction, despite giving precisely the same three dosages of pentylenetetrazol immediately after each day's session and having a range of ages of subjects. Meanwhile, Thiessen *et al.* (1961) and Calhoun (1965) sought to account for the facilitatory effects on memory for learned tasks of strychnine sulfate by demonstrating that it depressed activity (and hence reduced putatively interfering posttrial activity). In the first study cited, it was shown that mice of the C57BL/Crgl and the RIII/Crgl strains in fact showed depressed exploratory activity in response to 1.0 mg/kg as compared to saline-injected controls, and in the second, Calhoun demonstrated a comparable effect on home cage activity. In addition to the C57BL mice, as before, he used the C3H and the A strain, all in the Crgl sublines, and explored the effect of six doses, ranging from 0.2 to 1.2 mg/kg. Once again the C57BL mice showed the least activity overall but the dose–response curves did not differ from each other in their essentially parallel linearity, that is, there was no drug–strain interaction. Strychnine was also used by Karczmar and Scudder (1969) in their interesting interspecies comparisons, already cited (Chapter 2), but the main within-species comparisons used pemoline magnesium hydroxide. Several strains were represented among the mice from the *Mus musculus* species studied, including the C57BL/6 strain, along with the other species used, deermice and meadow voles. The complex apparatus (see Section 5.2) combined some of the features of a maze and of escape-avoidance conditioning, but the data were not reported in a form that allows a drug–strain interaction—as opposed to a drug–species interaction—to be accurately assessed. Study of the bar diagrams presented (their Figure 9-5) suggests that the intermediate dose used (3.0 mg/kg) had a possibly significant facilitatory effect on the three strains used with the larger dose (12.0 mg/kg) being on the average inhibitory with respect to a latency measure. But it is not clear from the account given whether the drug was administered before or after trials, so the bearing these results have on consolidation hypotheses must remain uncertain.

Wimer *et al.* (1968), on the other hand, clearly demonstrated a drug–strain interaction in the behavioral effects of etherization until mice lost the righting response and breathing became deep and irregular. They showed that such treatment, given immediately after learning trials, facilitated retention in both active- and passive-avoidance learning among the DBA/2J strain while not affecting that of the C57BL/6J mice. In further work, Wimer (1973) used different strains of mice, BDP/J and SJL/J, but noted the effects of posttrial etherization on active- and on passive-avoidance conditioning, respectively. This use of different tasks for the two strains vitiates the possibility of studying the drug–strain interaction further, though, reverting to the DBA and C57 strains, Wimer (1968) used reserpine to show that the latter strain could also show comparable facilitation by ether, if the learning trials of the active-avoidance task were preceded by intraperitoneal injections of 0.96 mg/kg of the drug. Reserpine was chosen for its known effects in depleting brain dopamine,

norepinephrine, and GABA, which are thus identified as possibly implicated in the previously reported stimulant effect on them of ether. Elias and
Simmerman (1971) followed Wimer's procedure of etherization but administered it to mice of the two strains both before and after 30 daily trials
in a spatial discrimination apparatus using escape from water as the motivation. Pretrial etherization yielded only an overall difference in swimming
speed and not errors, the treated subjects being *faster*, whereas posttrial
drug treatment showed a drug–strain interaction for both errors and speed
only when the stage of learning was considered. Thus while both strains
showed a decrement in performance, the C57BL/6J strain was the more affected. Unpublished data suggesting that this strain was also more sensitive
to ether, as compared to halothane anesthesia or an air blast, in reducing in-
centive to escape in the swimming situation were reported by Elias and
Pentz (1975, p. 252), along with others relating to work noted as by Elias *et
al.* and Simmerman *et al.* (their Table 4, pp. 246–247). The summary provided suggests that ether and halothane under certain conditions affect
neither strain, whereas under others, drug–strain interactions in learning the
spatial discrimination were detected, but the necessarily brief tabular details
do not allow further evaluation. A genetic analysis (Elias and Eleftheriou,
1975*a*) of strain differences in response to halothane anesthesia, using
the technique of recombinant inbred strains (see Chapter 8) is discussed
later.

Heinze (1974) also used ether with a passive-avoidance task, but with
three inbred strains of rats, and a selection of three of the possible six
F_1 crosses between them, a breeding design that constitutes a half-diallel
cross, for which appropriate analyses exist (Jones, 1965). Etherization to 15
sec beyond the loss of the righting response, given 15 min after one trial on
which shock was delivered on leaving the start compartment, markedly
reduced the latency to enter the compartment on retest 24 hr later, as compared with a nonetherized group. The analysis presented does no more than
indicate the presence of significant strain and hybrid differences overall:
The pairwise comparisons, which are possible from the means presented,
suggest heterosis in the response to ether.

Seiden and Peterson (1968) were concerned, on the other hand, with
the effect of reserpine as a depressant of performance in two-way avoidance
conditioning in DBA/1 and C57BL/10 mice as modified in turn by treatment with L-dopa, which acts as a behavioral antagonist to reserpine and
whose effect is consequently to restore performance temporarily. While the
effects of reserpine as such (2.5 mg/kg 20 hr prior to testing) were essentially identical in the two strains, there was some evidence that the time course

of the temporary recovery, occasioned by 400 mg/kg L-dopa given immediately before test trials of avoidance conditioning, varied between the strains. The C57 mice showed a briefer restoration of responding than the DBA mice, as seen in the number of successful avoidance responses, falling significantly below the DBA strain between 25 and 35 min after the start of the session. Other behavioral indices such as avoidance latencies and intertrial crossings from the escape–avoidance conditioning test show parallel results, though it is clear that the effect, which can itself be blocked in turn by a dopa-decarboxylase inhibitor, is not due solely to a restoration of activity as such by the L-dopa. Brain amine analysis shows a similar differential time course in the two strains, thus confirming the drug–strain interaction.

Injections of α-methyl-dopa in its racemic form after training in a Y-shaped discriminative avoidance apparatus of the kind used by Anisman (see Section 5.2) enabled Kitahama *et al.* (1975, 1976) to demonstrate a marked difference between C57BL/6 and C57BR/cd mice, both of the /Orl substrain. Administration of 100 mg/kg 24 hr before six daily test sessions effected a dramatic diminution in both number of avoidances and of correct responses in the latter strain, whereas the C57BL mice showed, on the contrary, a significant improvement in avoidances, though not in correct responding. The acute effects on performance of the same dose given to trained mice varied little between strains, and the effects on paradoxical sleep observed in EEG records obtained through implanted electrodes (see also Kitahama and Valatx, 1975) were essentially the same. These effects were relatively transitory, which excludes the possibility of drug-induced artifacts in locomotor responses 24 hr later being responsible for the interaction observed.

Following work by Randt *et al.* (1971) on passive-avoidance conditioning in C57BL/6J and DBA/2J mice, employing the protein synthesis inhibitor, cycloheximide, which disrupted learning on retest differentially when given 30 min before a single trial, depending on strain and test–retest interval, van Abeelen *et al.* (1973) also used cycloheximide to investigate its effect on three inbred strains of mice. All were injected subcutaneously with 50, 100, or 150 mg/kg prior to training to a criterion in black–white discrimination learning in a T-shaped water maze. Retention tests at 1- and 14-day intervals showed that mice of one strain, the DBA/2JNmg, had no retention loss, while others, the BA/Nmg (a cinnamon strain), retained nothing, not even the saline-control animals, which effectively eliminates the effect of cycloheximide. However, the C57BL/6JNmg mice showed a significant effect after 24 hr at the 100-mg/kg dose, 150 having proved toxic. These two studies show quite clearly that the amnesic effect of the drug is strain dependent, though the EEG, rather than behavioral responses to cycloheximide and also to diethyldithiocarbamide (a dopamine beta hydroxylase inhibitor) in the same two strains as before, reported by Randt *et al.* (1973), were probably based on insufficient numbers to demonstrate a strain difference. At least, none is mentioned.

In a similar investigatory rationale, Flood *et al.* (1974) used another protein synthesis inhibitor, anisomycin (2-*p*-methoxyphenyl-3-acetoxy-4-hydropryolidine) in conjunction with a passive-avoidance training situation, in which the retention of the experience of being shocked in a white compartment was tested 1 week after training under the effect of an injection (route not stated) of anisomycin of 0.5 mg/mouse. Among six strains, all inbred except for a random-bred Swiss strain, and including a C57BL/6J strain, no important strain differences were detected in the marked amnesic effect observed. Similarly, Appel (1965) found no difference between the latter strain and CF white mice in degree of inhibition of RNA synthesis occasioned by actomycin D. It is unfortunate therefore that Flood *et al.* dropped the DBA/2J strain because of training difficulties; but even without this strain, the lack of confirmation of van Abeelen's and Randt *et al.*'s earlier findings is apparent and reasons must presumably be sought in differences in the postulated mode of action of the protein synthesis inhibitors used in the two studies.

The effect on avoidance conditioning of *p*-chlorophenylalanine, which in addition to being a brain-serotonin depletor depresses the hydroxylating capacities of the liver with respect to phenylalanine and tryptophan, was investigated by Schlesinger *et al.* (1968a) using the DBA/2J and C57BL/6J strains of mice. A clear facilitatory effect of chronic administration of the drug (320 mg/kg per day from birth to testing at 21 days) on both learning and resistance to extinction of avoidance responding was shown, without, however, evidence of a drug–strain interaction. A similar regimen applied to rats of the Buffalo and Fischer strains failed to affect their conditioned pole-jumping response markedly, but in an experiment in which a single injection (same dosage) was given orally 3 days before the same test a strain difference in favor of the Fischer strain rats was shown, though once again this difference did not interact with *p*-chlorophenylalanine.

The segment of the work on drugs affecting animals' sensitivity to convulsions and their acquisition and/or retention of learned tasks that we have chosen to review is, of course, only that part of a larger whole that is concerned with hereditary determination. A summary will be found in Table XII. Clearly, drug–strain interactions are implicated, but our survey contains little by way of breeding designs, which could lead to a more precise evaluation and specifically to indications of the genetical architecture of the drug responses involved. Heinze's (1974) work comes nearest to approaching this desideratum.

Finally, concerning depressants, especially responses of the more behavioral kind—apart from alcohol, which will be considered later in the context of alcohol preference phenotypes and the like—the relevant literature is by contrast sparse. Vesell (1968) reports a thorough investigation of the effects of hexobarbital on sleep time in no less than 15 mouse strains, mostly inbred ones, and crosses between three of them (DBA/2N, AL/N, and BALB/c), which in fact constitute a partial 3 × 3 diallel cross. There is some evidence of drug–strain interaction in that the first two of the strains mentioned above, together with a C57BL/6N group, all had significantly longer sleep times than the rest, including the BALB/c mice, in response to a standard intraperitoneal injection of 125 mg/kg of sodium hexobarbital. The crossbreeds' results, while incompletely reported in detail, showed no evidence of obvious phenotypic dominance for either high or low scores. The greater sensitivity of males to barbiturates was confirmed and some evidence presented that relates the extent of this sex difference to the extent of inbreeding within the strains. The degree of variability evident within even highly inbred strains suggests some residual heterozygosity among the genes contributing to the determination of the sleep-time phenotype.

In summary, therefore, it is clear that the range and expertise of work on inbred strains in the mouse is equal if not superior to that on the rat. The relative lack of strains derived from selection experiments for behavioral or other characteristics, which figured so largely in our review of rat work, is amply compensated for by the energetic utilization of often quite large numbers of different mouse strains, well chosen for the differences they display with respect to behavioral or other traits of interest to psychopharmacology. A few such strains and their derivatives, such as the C57BL and DBA strains, have attained the status of standard strains in this and other areas of psychology [see, for example, the table provided by Mandel *et al.* (1974)], a conclusion that may be reinforced by descriptions of further work using them in what follows.

This then ends our review of work on the pharmacogenetics of inbred strains, except, first, for phenotypes relating to alcohol effects, including preference and dependence, which will be dealt with separately and, second, for a group of studies which are of considerable interest since they claim to have identified major gene effects governing behavior in the mouse, in-

TABLE XII

Psychopharmacogenetic Experiments with Convulsants, Anticonvulsants, and Amnesics

Reference	Species (and strain)	Drug	Measure	Outcome	Remarks
Busnel and Lehmann (1961)	Mice, Swiss albinos seizure prone and resistant	Cardiazol, strychnine, and caffeine (macrodose)	Seizure threshold	Dose response differences found	
Plotnikoff (1960, 1963b)	Mice, Swiss albino, DBA/1	Chlorpromazine	Seizure threshold	DBAs protected against seizure	
		Meprobamate		Drug–strain interaction	
		Reserpine		Drug–strain interaction	
	Heterogeneous	Chlorpromazine		Drug effect. No interaction	
				Protected against seizure	Progressive diminution of protection with inbreeding
Plotnikoff (1963a) Schlesinger and Griek (1970), Schlesinger et al. (1968a)	Mice, as above Mice, DBA/2 C57BL/6J, and F₁ crosses	Various drugs Reserpine Tetrabenazine	Preseizure running Seizure threshold	No interaction Lowered especially among DBAs	
		α-Methyl tyrosine		C57s resistant. DBAs and hybrids affected	DBA–C57BL strain differences quite robust
		p-Chlorphenylalanine 5-Hydroxytryptophan		No interaction Generally protective	
		Serotonin and norepinephrine Iproniazid		No interaction Protect inbreds but not crosses	
		Amino-oxyacetic acid		Protection from chemical seizure	
				F₁ crosses again unresponsive to protection from chemical seizure	Relevant to major gene coat-color differences?

Reference	Strains	Drug	Task	Results	Comments
Schlesinger et al. (1968b)	Mice, DBA, C57BL	Pentylenetetrazol	Seizure threshold (electrical induction)	Lowered especially among DBAs. No interaction	DBA–C57BL strain differences quite robust
Kitahama et al. (1975, 1976)	Mice, C57BL/6, C57BR/cd	α-Methyl-dopa	Y-discriminative avoidance	Reduced avoidance in C57BR Drug–strain interaction	
Kitahama and Valatx (1975)	Mice, C57BL/6, C57BR/cd	α-Methyl-dopa	Paradoxical sleep (EEG)	No interaction	
Randt et al. (1971)	Mice, C57BL/6J, DBA/2J	Cycloheximide	Passive avoidance	Learning disrupted Drug–strain interaction	
van Abeelen et al. (1973)	Mice, C57BL/6JNmg, DBA/2Nmg, NA/Nmg	Cycloheximide	T-discriminative avoidance	Drug–strain interaction	
Randt et al. (1973)	Mice, C57BL/6J, DAB/2J	Cycloheximide Diethyldithiocarbamide	EEG response	Strains not compared	Numbers small
Flood et al. (1974)	Mice, 6 strains including C57BL/6J	Anisomycin	Passive avoidance (shock amnesia)	No strain difference found	
Appel (1965)	Mice, C57BL, CF	Actomycin D	Inhibition of RNA synthesis	No strain difference found	
Schlesinger et al. (1968a)	Mice, C57BL/6J, DBA/2J	p-Chlorphenylalanine	Avoidance learning and extinction	Facilitates learning and resistance to extinction No interaction	
	Rats, Fischer, Buffalo	p-Chlorphenylalanine	Pole jumping	No effect, administered chronically or acutely	
Vesell (1968)	Mice, 15 strains and crosses	Sodium hexobarbital	Sleep time	Drug–strain interaction DBA, AL, and C57 all longer sleep time. Sex differences, male > female	Partial 3 × 3 diallel cross
Boggan and Seiden (1971)	Mice, DBA/2, DBA/1	Reserpine L-Dopa	Seizure threshold	Lowered Protected	
Bovet and Oliverio (1973), Oliverio (1974b)	Mice, SEC/1ReJ, DBA/2J, C57BL/6J, and crosses	Various	Seizure threshold	DBA and SEC lowered Drug–strain interaction	

(Continued)

TABLE XII—*Continued*

Reference	Species (and strain)	Drug	Measure	Outcome	Remarks
Meier et al. (1963)	Mice, 4 strains	Pentylenetetrazol	Seizure threshold	C57BL most resistant	
Bourgault et al. (1963)	Mice, C57BL/6J, SC-I	Pentylenetetrazol	Seizure threshold	Little strain difference	
		Pentobarbital Pentobarbital sodium	Activity	DBA/2 most protected Significant strain difference reversed	
		Reserpine	Activity	More reduced in low-scoring C57s	
Davis and Webb (1963, 1964), Davis and King (1967)	Mice, up to 6 strains	Flurothyl	Seizure threshold	Clear drug-strain interaction. DBA more susceptible than C57 and BALB	
Boggan et al. (1971)	Mice, C57BL/6, HS	5-Hydroxytryptophan	Seizure threshold after priming	Lowered. No interaction with strain	
Maxson et al. (1975)	Mice, C57BL, DBA	Amino-oxyacetic acid	Seizure threshold after priming	Drug prevents priming of C57s. Drug-strain interaction	
		Cycloheximide	Seizure threshold after priming	Drug prevents priming of C57s. Drug-strain interaction	
Yanai and Ginsburg (1973), Yanai et al. (1975)	Mice, C57BL, DBA, and crosses	Ethanol (chronic intake)	Seizure threshold	Lowered for offspring. C57 more than DBA. Cross-fostering proves postnatal effect	Firm basis for further analysis of these phenotypes
Krivanek and McGaugh (1968)	Mice, C57BL/6, BALB/c	Pentylenetetrazol	Lashley III maze	Generally facilitative. Low dose optimum for C57s. Drug-strain interaction	

Reference	Strain	Drug	Task	Result
Buckholtz (1974)	Mice, DBA/2J, C57BL/6J	Pentylenetetrazol	Shuttle box escape	No interaction
Thiessen et al. (1961)	Mice, C57BL/Crgl, RIII/Crgl	Strychnine sulfate	Exploration	Depressed
Calhoun (1965)	Mice, C57BL/Crgl, C3H/Crgl, A/Crgl	Strychnine sulfate	Home-cage activity	C57BL least active No interaction
Karczmar and Scudder (1969)	Mice, including C57BL, deermice, meadow voles	Pemoline Mg hydroxide	Escape-avoidance maze	Interaction not assessable from data
Wimer et al. (1968)	Mice, C57BL/6J, DBA/2J	Ether	Active and passive avoidance learning	Drug–strain interaction DBA facilitated. C57 facilitated after reserpine priming
Wimer (1973)	Mice, BDP/J, SJL/J	Ether	Active and passive avoidance separately	Interaction not assessable from method
Elias and Simmerman (1971)	Mice, including C57BL/6J	Ether	Discrimination learning (water escape)	Increased swimming speed (pretrial treatment). Drug–strain interactions (posttrial treatment)
Elias and Pentz (1975)	Mice, including C57BL	Ether	Swimming escape	Reduced escape incentive—C57s most affected Drug–strain interaction
Heinze (1974)	Rats, 3 strains and crosses	Halothane Ether	Passive avoidance	Reduced latency Heterosis suggested
Seiden and Peterson (1968)	Mice, DBA/1, C57BL/10	Reserpine + L-dopa	Two-way avoidance	Reserpine similar for strains, L-dopa acts shorter on C57s than on DBAs. Clear drug–strain interaction

cluding some specifically relating to drug responses. The technique employed is that of recombinant inbred strains, and some attention must be paid to the origin of this technique insofar as it relates to present concerns.

Chapter 8

Recombinant Inbred Strains

The flurry of interest in the literature in the use of recombinant inbred strains for the analysis of behavioral inheritance appears to stem from the work of Bailey (1971) at the Jackson Laboratory at Bar Harbor, Maine. In this influential paper he was, however, concerned not with behavioral phenotypes but rather with histocompatibility as evidenced by skin graft rejection and, to a minor extent, with coat color. Recombinant inbred or RI strains are created by the technique of repeated inbreeding over successive generations, in order to fix genetically the variation resulting from recombination. It is a familiar technique in genetics and has also been used in psychogenetics (van Abeelen, 1970). Recombination is essentially the process, seen, for example, in segregation in an F_2 population derived from a cross of inbred strains, which results in progeny that differ from their parents in their individual combination of genes. It is also the mechanism by which the genes of the progeny of a randomly breeding population come to be different from those of their parents.

However, what is novel in this approach based on recombination is the use of RI strains in conjunction with a series of congenic lines developed by repeated backcrossing to one of the two parental mouse strains, the C57BL/6By, so that each congenic strain differs from this strain only by an introduced chromosomal segment carrying the other BALB/cBy strain allele at a distinctive histocompatibility locus. Testing each of these congenic lines in turn against each of the seven RI strains used* indicates, by means of the reaction to skin grafts on RI × C57BL F_1 hosts, whether or

---

*It is reported that four other series of recombinant inbred strains involving five additional progenitor strains are being developed (Taylor, 1976).

not that RI strain carries the BALB allele and hence leads to graft survival, as opposed to the C57BL strain, which occasions rejection. In this way what is termed a "*strain distribution pattern*" or SDP is built up for each locus, and matching SDPs, excluding, as seems reasonable, chance occurrence ($p = 2^{-7} = 1/128 = 0.0078$), therefore indicate identity or close linkage.

Bailey and Hoste's application (1971) to the problem of the detection of a female immune response in mice seems satisfactory, based as it is on the direct observation of skin graft survival, though it should perhaps be noted that "One unexpected exceptional rejection of a female graft was deemed likely to be attributable to a mutation" (p. 405). But with the extension to other, especially behavioral, phenotypes comes the problem of typing essentially quantitative variables—the classic problem in the application of Mendelian analyses to continuous variation. The conceptual gap is hardly bridged by Bailey's (1971) brief reference to data on three coat-color loci, since the manner of obtaining the strain distribution patterns for them is not explained. Presumably progeny testing was involved.

The first application to the quantitative area reported was, however, not concerned with behavior but rather with the amount of serotonin circulating in the blood, for which the C57BL and BALB strains differ markedly (Eleftheriou and Bailey, 1972*a*). The analysis fell out very neatly, both reciprocal crosses and three of the recombinant strains having values not significantly different from the C57BL and the other four similarly resembling the BALB strain, together with one of the congenic lines which, moreover, had a strain distribution pattern identical with the distribution of the serotonin phenotypes. This latter fact was established, presumably by skin grafting to RI-derived hosts, though this is not explicitly stated in this short paper. On the basis of this evidence a single dominant autosomal gene, linked, in a group as yet unknown, to the histocompatibility locus discovered in the congenic line, was claimed to have been identified and the symbol *Spl* was proposed, with the superscript *h* to designate the allele determining the high level of systemic serotonin and *l* for that determining the low.

In a similar vein is a study of blood corticosterone levels by Eleftheriou and Bailey (1972*b*), though the SDP analysis was not mentioned in this connection. Instead, this is a straightforward study of the phenotypic values for the parental, reciprocal crosses and RI strains, augmented in a second experiment with both the usual backcrosses and two crosses between the C57BL parental strain and two of the RI strains. The latter yielded values used to support arguments about the similarity and dissimilarity of the strains involved in the crosses. But it was on the backcross data that much of the subsequent interpretation rests, since in both cases they gave distributions that were shown by statistical techniques, whose validity it would seem difficult to deny, to be bimodal. The phenotypic values fall precisely, therefore, into four groups, having phenotypic values of roughly 4 units (low), 8 (intermediate, including the B_1 high and the B_2 low groupings), 12 (high), and 16 (heterotic). These four phenotypes encouraged the authors to postulate a two-gene model, symbolized by *Cpl-1* and *Cpl-2*, governing circulating (that is, resting) corticosterone levels, with superscripts *h* and *l* as before indicating the alleles at the two loci determining the high and low levels, respectively. No linkage data were, of course, offered, the congenic strains not having been used. A similar approach was adopted in a further study by Eleftheriou (1974) in which the corticosterone content of the brain in the two parental strains was assessed by measurement of radioactive uptake by the hypothalamus 40 min after the injection of a labeled dose of the hormone. Marked differences between the progenitor strains with respect to this steroid-binding process were reported, the BALB group having a significantly lower count. Reciprocal and backcrosses, together with crosses to the RI strain gave results that did not, however, match any strain distribution pattern, so that no more can be done than to make the assumption that the process is controlled by at least one genetic locus, a conclusion with which it would be hard to disagree.

In the next papers offered by this group, Oliverio *et al.* (1973*b*) began consideration of psychological phenotypes, in this case two-way escape–avoidance conditioning. The now familiar genetic approach was used to analyze scores for each strain and cross based on the performance in the shuttle box during five consecutive daily sessions of 50 trials each, the actual metric being the improvement between day 1 and day 5. On day 1 there were no significant differences between the strains, whereas by day 5 two (only) highly significantly different groupings had developed. Three of the recombinant strains together with the parental BALB strain gave high scores, whereas the other four RIs, both of the reciprocals, and the C57BL gave low scores. Also giving low scores was a congenic line having a strain distribution pattern that matched that of the recombinant inbreds, from which the authors concluded that, despite this match, "active avoidance performance (presumably *high* performance) is not linked to (the histocompatibility gene carried by the congenic strain in question)" (p. 498). Rather, they focus attention on another congenic strain that does have a high, BALB-like performance, but which breaks the strain distribution pattern of the recombinant inbreds in one case only, where it has the BALB histocompatibility allele, whereas the recombinant strain in question has the C57BL and, moreover, resembles the C57 in having a low-avoidance performance in this experiment. This and other considerations lead the authors to conclude that lower performance was determined by a single dominant autosomal gene, linked to that carried by the second congenic line on chromosome 9 in linkage group II, and proposed *Aal* as the designation with the same superscript conventions as before. They note the possible connection with serotonin determination, since the congenic line in question was the one referred to by Eleftheriou and Bailey (1972*a*), but do not comment on the fact that the linkage group now appears to have been discovered. They also note the support to be derived for their formulation from other work, including Wilcock's reanalysis (1969) of Collins' diallel data (1964) in which Wilcock showed that the placement of the (same) BALB strain on the diallel covariance–variance diagram he plotted was such as to suggest extreme recessivity, in contrast to the tight grouping of the other four strains used, which included the (same) C57 strain, and speculated on the involvement of a single recessive. Applications of the recombinant inbred method to various other aspects of mouse behavior, with varying degrees of success, are summarized in Table XIII and include those reported for water escape (Elias and Eleftheriou, 1975*b*), maze learning (Oliverio *et al.*, 1975*a*), ovulation in response to noise or light (Eleftheriou and Kristal, 1974), aggressiveness, wheel running, and testosterone levels (Lucas and Eleftheriou, 1975; Eleftheriou *et al.*, 1976), dominance behavior (Messeri *et al.*, 1975), activity and brain epinephrine (Moisset, 1977). Work is included on analgesia (Shuster *et al.*, 1975*b*; Oliverio *et al.*, 1975*b*; Baran *et al.*, 1975), which will be discussed later (see Section 9.2). Mention may also be made of additional work by Eleftheriou *et al.* (1974) on aggression as measured by isolation-induced fighting among these same strains, which is remarkable for the suggestion of a cytoplasmic effect (see Section 9.2) on a behavioral character.

This preamble allows us to consider papers extending this approach to psychopharmacogenetics. However, Oliverio *et al.* (1973*a*) also dealt with a behavioral phenotype unmodified by the influence of a drug and this was crossing activity as recorded automatically in a two-compartment activity or toggle cage during ten minutes. Results for this basal exploratory activity, so called since it was measured after not a drug but a saline control injection, showed that the strains and crosses fell into two reasonably distinct (and significantly different) groups with the BALB parental and three recombinants in the low and the C57BL, the reciprocals, and the other four recombinants in the high group, which also contained the high-scoring group of the bimodally distributed backcross to the BALB, differentiated statistically as before (Eleftheriou and Bailey, 1972*b*). The low group contained the rest of the recombinant inbred distribution and a congenic strain that closely matched the recombinant strain distribution pattern. On this basis, supported by cited results in the literature from the work of their own group and others, they postulated the *Exa* gene, linked to the histocompatibility gene on chromosome 4 in linkage group VIII. Extension of this approach to the multivariate definition of exploration as contrasted with activity is anticipated (Simmel, 1976). Of the two drugs employed in this study, the results for amphetamine proved unamenable to analysis by the methods described in that the dose–response curves fell into no simple groupings—there being six in all—and it is concluded "that the modification of basal activity by d-amphetamine is due to a polygenic effect which is highly complex to analyze genetically. For this reason, no further genetic testing was pursued for this effect" (Oliverio *et al.*, 1973*a*, p. 897). But for scopolamine greater success in the application of this methodology is reported: Strains were differentiated with respect to the kind of dose–response curve they displayed, that is, persistently decreasing their activity in response to increasing dosages (three in all) as did the C57BL, both reciprocals, and three of the recombinant inbred strains, persistently increasing (the BALB and two more recombinants), or maintaining the same response after an initial increase to the lowest dose (the remaining two recombinants). The genetic reasoning followed is so complex that it is best to let the authors speak for themselves on the subject. "To arrive at the genetic basis for the plateau effect. . . , (two) congenic lines. . . were tested since both carry the BALB/cBy chromosomal segment which includes the (histocompatibility) locus with a (strain distribution pattern) matching that of the scopolamine effect. One line was BALB/cBY-like; the other was not. This result indicates that (the histocompatibility locus cited) itself is not directly involved in this effect, but only that the locus for non-progressive response to scopolamine is probably linked to (it)" (p. 896). And further, ". . . the confirmation by the use of (the two) congenic lines. . . indicating that this effect is not a pleiotropic effect of the (cited) locus although it is probably closely linked to it. The lack of a plateauing effect in the BALB/c strain which also carried (the same histocompatibility locus) can only be explained by yet other modifier gene(s) in BALB/c background" (p. 898). On this seemingly slender evidence the symbol *Sco* is proposed for a gene linked to the locus cited in chromosome 17 of linkage group IX "which controls the sustained reactivity to scopolamine once the initial response has occurred, the other allele permitting reversal of exploratory activity determined at *Exa*" (p. 898). Superscripts *a* for absent and *p* for present are added.

The effects of chlorpromazine are similarly analyzed in another paper (Castellano *et al.*, 1974), and though the phenotype being modified here is avoidance conditioning of the same kind used in the group's analysis of its genetic determinants (Oliverio *et al.*, 1973*b*), drug–response considerations are again paramount. After training to reach criterion performance, which confirmed the relative standings of the strains as reported before, the changes caused by four different dose levels (1.0, 1.5, 2.0, and 4.0 mg/kg) on individual performances were measured. All declined, but the dose–response curves varied as before, some being progressive and others changing little, as between the third and fourth doses. The parental strains

TABLE XIII

Major Gene Analysis of Various Phenotypes in Inbred Strains of Mice
Using Recombinant Inbreds (RI) and Strain Distribution Patterns (SDP)[a]

Reference	Measure	Genetic Technique	Outcome	Remarks
Bailey and Hoste (1971)	Immune response	RI, SDP	Dominant gene governing early response	
Eleftheriou and Bailey (1972)	Plasma serotonin level	RI, SDP	Locus *Spl* identified	
Eleftheriou and Bailey (1972b)	Plasma corticosterone level	RI only	Loci *Cpl-1* and *Cpl-2*	No linkage
Oliverio et al. (1973b)	Escape–avoidance conditioning	RI, SDP	Locus *Aal*	
Oliverio et al. (1973a)	Exploratory activity	RI, SDP	Locus *Exa*	
	Exploratory activity under amphetamine	RI only	No coherent pattern	Probably polygenic
	Exploratory activity under scopolamine	RI, SDP	Locus *Sco*	
Castellano et al. (1974)	Escape–avoidance conditioning under chlorpromazine	RI, SDP	Locus *Cpz*	
Messeri et al. (1975)	Social dominance	RI only	3 unspecified loci	
Eleftheriou et al. (1974)	Aggression	RI, SDP	Cytoplasmic effect?	
Lucas and Eleftheriou (1975)	Plasma testosterone level	RI only		Some relation to aggression

Reference	Character		Comment	
Oliverio and Eleftheriou (1976)	Activity after ethanol	RI, SDP	Locus *Eam*	
Elias and Eleftheriou (1975a)	Halothane anesthesia	RI only	No coherent pattern	Parental strains not different
Oliverio et al. (1975a)	Maze learning	RI only	No coherent pattern	Probably polygenic
Baran et al. (1975)	Opiate receptors	RI only	No coherent pattern	Probably polygenic
	Morphine analgesia	RI only	No analysis attempted	
Shuster (1975), Shuster et al. (1975b)	Pain response	RI, SDP	No locus identifiable	
	Morphine analgesia	RI only	No coherent pattern	
	Activity after morphine	RI, SDP	No locus identifiable	Probably polygenic?
Oliverio et al. (1975b)	Activity after morphine	RI, SDP	No analysis attempted	Probably polygenic
	Morphine analgesia	RI only	No coherent pattern	
	Morphine tolerance	RI, SDP	Major gene linkage possible	
Eleftheriou et al. (1976)	Wheel-running activity	RI, SDP	No coherent pattern	
Elias and Eleftheriou (1975b)	Water escape	RI, SDP	Locus *Bfo*	Albino gene not involved
Eleftheriou and Kristal (1974)	Ovulation to bell or flash	RI, SDP	Possible locus	
Moisset (1977)	Cerebral norepinephrine	RI, SDP		
	Open-field ambulation	RI, SDP		
Eleftheriou (1974)	Hypothalamic norepinephrine	RI, SDP	Major gene, not identifiable	
Eleftheriou (1975a)	Male pheromone	RI, SDP	Locus *Phr*	

aBased, in part, on a table from Eleftheriou (1975a).

were not especially sharply differentiated in terms of their responses, which was presumably why the authors, while stressing the maximal efficiency of the methods used when the progenitor strains differed significantly, argued the utility of strain distribution patterns matching even when they do not. Thus they prepared the ground for the use of two of the RI strains that showed the extremes of response at nearly all drug doses as the standard strains against which to evaluate the distribution patterns of two congenic strains, in contrast to previous practice. In one case the congenic strain's response (to one dose only of chlorpromazine) resembled the extreme recombinant strain's value, and the location of one gene in a two-gene model was claimed as confirmed—despite the discrepancy of one mismatch in the SDP for the locus putatively governing the response to that dose*—whereas in the other case, despite a perfect match of the strain distribution pattern with the other dose, the congenic strain showed an in-termediate performance unlike that of the recombinant strain at the other extreme of that dose response, and the location of the second gene was declared unconfirmed. It is not clear what is the reasoning behind these deductions, especially since the BALB parental strain is also similarly in-termediate, but it probably lies in the complexities of the two-gene model that the authors present. Nevertheless they proposed a *Cpz* gene on chromosome 9, linkage group II, with superscript *a* for the BALB strain allele for low and *b* for the C57BL allele for high avoidance after chlor-promazine. The similarity of the location proposed for the *Aal* gene was not commented on.

Finally, consideration must be given to a study of the effects of alcohol on activity in the mouse. Oliverio and Eleftheriou (1976) used the same technique as described above for mensuration, and administered the drug at four dose levels (0.5, 1.0, 1.5, and 2.0 g/kg) intraperitoneally 10 min before the single 20-min test in the two-compartment activity box. A saline control group for each of the strains and crosses enabled a comparison with the saline control group from the previous experiment (Oliverio *et al.*, 1973*a*), the rank orders for which correlated $+0.81$, an impressive value when it is considered that the test period was twice as long. Under alcohol, all activity scores declined and further consideration of them was made in terms of the percentage decline in scores. Thus, the change score or a direct measure of response to the drug was now the phenotype. These values ex-hibited two clear groupings: The C57BL and two RI strains showed a relatively large decline approaching 80%–90% of saline (control) activity at the largest dose (2.0 g/kg), while all the other strains showed more modest responses. The other progenitor strain, the BALB, had the average value

---

*A misprint in the table must be suspected here, since the text explicitly claims a match.

for this group, which was a decline of about 45% from saline control values. Several congenic strains having matched SDPs, for the distribution of C57 versus BALB histocompatibility loci were tested under the same conditions, with the outcome that one had scores resembling the C57BL strain for activity under ethanol. This major gene effect was regarded as confirmed by a bimodality in the distribution of scores of a backcross. The locus thus identified was on the same chromosome 4 (linkage group VIII) as that labeled as *Exa*, governing undrugged activity, but is not identical to it since a different congenic strain is involved. The authors therefore postulated the *Eam* (*e*thanol *a*ctivity *m*odifier) gene, with *Eam^h* for the allele for high-activity decline, as seen in the C57 phenotype, and *Eam^l* for low-activity decline as in the BALB.

Other papers using this methodology that are of psychopharmacogenetic interest will be considered later in the appropriate context, but a summary of the findings at hand at the time of writing is presented in Table XIII. One, however, by Elias and Eleftheriou (1975*a*) relates to a phenotype of primarily pharmacological rather than behavioral interest, though the connection between research on anesthetics and the topic of memory consolidation has been emphasized by, for example, Elias and Pentz (1975) and renders it of sufficient behavioral relevance to be considered here. Using three concentrations (2%, 3%, and 4%) of halothane anesthesia, the times to induce the loss of righting reflexes were determined under precisely controlled conditions and the time to their recovery was also obtained. For neither measure under any of the three dosages used was there a sufficiently clear statistical differentiation between any of the progenitor, F_1 and the seven RI strains to allow comparison of the strain distribution patterns with congenic lines to identify major gene loci. Polygenic determination must be suspected, therefore, but it should be noted that, in the absence of significant differences between the progenitor C57BL and BALB strains, at least in recovery times to halothane anesthesia, no genetic analysis is likely to prove fruitful since the essential basis of significant strain differences is lacking. The time-to-induction measure shows more promise, the C57BL strain being more susceptible than the other, the BALB, or their reciprocal crosses, with significantly shorter induction times at all three concentrations. The absence, in contrast, of any significant differences between the other three strains mentioned, points to the absence of prenatal maternal influences, as the authors note, and to a degree of potence (phenotypic dominance) that is probably complete.

A review paper by Oliverio (1974*a*) offered an evaluation of this Italo-American research endeavor. After discussion of morphological evolution, especially in relation to brain size, Oliverio turns to psychogenetics and reviews the work of his colleagues on the mouse, which he argues constitutes the material of choice, including studies using selection, mutants, and some biometrical techniques, before turning to the "recent and more refined method of genetic analysis based on the strain distribution pattern in a set of recombinant inbred strains. . ." (Oliverio, 1974*a*, p. 15). No very strong claims are made for the primacy of this methodology and the review closes with a brief account of some human studies with an emphasis on linkages in connection with blood groups, color blindness, and depressive psychosis. Further accounts and appraisals of the methodology were provided by Eleftheriou (1975*a*), Oliverio (1974*b*), Oliverio and Castellano (1975), and by Eleftheriou and Elias (1975), who also presented correlational data of RI strain scores on several tests under a range of dosages of several drugs. The descriptive analyses employed are no more than suggestive of genotype–environment interactions and, as the authors recognize, are no substitute for thorough genetic analysis.

While it is clear that the work surveyed in this section can be criticized on several grounds, there is no gainsaying that it adds up to an impressive programmatic effort. The behavioral techniques employed are always adequate and usually quite sophisticated. The statistical analyses, though generally rather cursorily reported, are well chosen and appropriately powerful. There is some measure of replication of a supportive kind, both internally and from earlier work and other workers, most of which was featured in this book. Perhaps more congenic strains were screened for distribution patterns than were reported in the final matches and near matches, and indeed, as much was admitted with commendable candor when this approach failed. But it is, of course, with respect to the basic proposition that major genes that govern behavioral responses to situations and to drugs have been identified in the mouse that the impact must be evaluated, and here the edifice of interpretation that has been erected creaks. I have indicated above the places where this seems to me to have been the case; doubtless there are others (Klein, 1977).

Turning to the more general problem in genetics of the identification of major gene loci, attempts along not dissimilar lines have a long history. Jinks and Pooni (1976) provided a generalized treatment of predictive possibilities in plant material. Evaluation of the current attempt using behavioral phenotypes is therefore best left to geneticists, but a recent paper is helpful in this connection in providing an illustration that also comes from plant genetics. Eaves and Brumpton (1972) used 82 out of no less than 100 recombinant inbred lines of the tobacco plant established by selfing F_2s, the total that survived to F_8 (or F_7 only in 13% of them). As part of a large study primarily concerned with the identification by multivariate techniques of the covariation—genetical, environmental, and interactional—of factors governing such phenotypic aspects of the plant as flowering time, size of leaf, etc., they investigated the number of effective factors, that is, genes or groups of genes acting together, likely to account for the variation observed. Estimates range from between two and four for early height to seven to ten for plant diameter. They comment, "The values obtained for the number of effective factors suggest that sufficient loci are involved in the variation to make identification of individual gene effects impracticable" (p. 169). Attempts to group the lines by statistical techniques of considerably greater sophistication than those used in the mouse work reviewed confirmed the need to postulate "a large number of effective factors to account for the observed variation" (p. 170). One interesting suggestion to emerge from this work is the strong hint that two independent sets of genes, probably operative at different stages in the plant's growth, are implicated—a conclusion strongly reminiscent of the situation demonstrated to exist in the acquisition of escape–avoidance conditioning in the rat (Wilcock and Fulker, 1973), and which might well be proposed as a not unlikely mechanism involved in the response by an organism to drugs, or even to different sizes of dose of the same drug. This notion seems to be a not implausible alternative to the simple genetical determination of drug response claimed to have been demonstrated by the Rome–Bar Harbor group. Another might be the so-called buffering mechanism shown by Fulker (1970) to have some generality of operation in rodent response to stress, including, be it noted, that of the plasma corticosteroid in mice, the *resting* determination of which was claimed by Eleftheriou and Bailey (1972*b*) to be rather simply determined in the mouse.

Further evaluation must follow, but it is beyond the scope of this monograph to attempt it. In particular, the validity of the particular models suggested can be assessed by internal evidence relating to the biometrical genetical model, which they imply, and the extent to which they prove consistent with the parameters of such models. Preliminary investigations along these lines suggest that the fit is not always within an acceptable range.

In summary, this chapter has reviewed part of the basis for the claims to have located in the laboratory mouse, by the use of recombinant inbred strains and the technique of matching strain distribution patterns of congenic marker strains, genes governing psychopharmacological and behavioral responses. Aspects of this considerable body of work, which induce caution in evaluating these claims, are highlighted.

tion affecting this phenotype is suspected. An alternative mechanism, genetic drift, is invoked to account for the instability of preference differences between inbred strains not of mice but of rats from different dealers (Wise, 1974), but the obvious possibility of husbandry, that is, environmental, differences would need to be excluded before such a claim could be entertained.

Anisman and Waller (1974) incidentally reported the absence of any strain difference between male rats of the Sprague–Dawley and Holtzman strains in the development of a preference for 7.9% (wt./vol.) alcohol over water after a series of inescapable shocks. Amit *et al.* (1976) showed that Sprague–Dawleys and Wistars responded similarly to alcohol, either ingested voluntarily or injected, in ways that allowed the conclusion that the action of disulfiram as an antialcoholic was based largely on its inhibition of dopamine beta hydroxylase. But the work of the greatest saliency in connection with the determination of strain differences in preference in the rat was that of Melchior and Myers (1976), who used the same two strains, plus two others, the Long–Evans and the Wistar. Pursuing the hypothesis that the pattern of ethanol preference may be the outcome of a functional imbalance in the activity of monoamines in the central nervous system, they sought to manipulate the serotonergic and catecholaminergic systems directly by biochemical intervention. In this they based themselves on work such as that of Ahtee and Eriksson (1973), who showed (see Chapter 3) that the latter's AA strain, selected for high alcohol preference, had higher brain serotonin than the low-preference strain (ANA) and their own findings (Myers and Melchior, 1975) that dietary manipulation by means of excess tryptophan, which raises brain serotonin level, could augment preference. But the effect they found in that work was strain dependent: Of the two strains common to both studies, only one, male Long–Evans rats, responded with increased ethanol intake to L-tryptophan dietary concentrations of 1% and 3% (by weight), whereas the Sprague–Dawleys, a generally low-preference strain, showed no significant effect in either sex when presented with increasing concentrations of ethanol (2.4%–23.7% wt./vol.) over a 12-day experiment. This finding was in considerable contrast to rats of an altogether different strain, known as Royal Victoria, not listed as an inbred strain by Festing and Staats (1973). Females of this hooded strain, a higher preference strain as compared with Sprague–Dawleys, responded significantly, showing a considerable elevation in intake in response to the 3% tryptophan, especially at concentrations below 11.9% (wt./vol.). It was perhaps unfortunate therefore that this strain was not included in the four which, as noted above, were used for the later experiment, in which direct intracerebral injection techniques were used to assess effects on preference, measured in the same way as before. Lesions in the serotonergic system were created by acute intraventricular injections in appropriate doses of

5,6-dihydroxytryptamine (5,6-DHT) and in the catecholaminergic system
by 6-hydroxydopamine (6-OHDA), control animals, matched with respect to
alcohol preference, being injected with an artificial cerebrospinal fluid. The
effectiveness of these treatments was monitored by regional brain assays of
the levels of serotonin, norepinephrine, and dopamine, though in the
Sprague–Dawley strain only. Additionally, injections of 5,7-dihydroxy-
tryptamine (5,7-DHT) were also employed to deplete brain serotonin and
norepinephrine, but in only three of the four strains under comparison, the
Sprague–Dawleys, the Wistars, and the Holtzmans, the Long-Evans rats
being omitted in this case. Thus the measures of alcohol preference were
taken before the pharmacological intervention, 10 days and 60 days after it.
The outcomes were fairly clear cut, and indicated an important drug–strain
interaction in the way the neurotoxins employed affected behavior, which
may be summarized by noting that the 5,6-DHT treatment increased
preference to some extent in all strains except the Wistar where it had no effect, whereas the 6-OHDA decreased preference generally, except in the
Holtzman strain where it had little or no effect. Thus the Sprague–Dawley
strain stood out as being sensitive to *both* treatments in a way not evident
for other strains. 5,7-DHT did not affect preference in the three strains used
for this treatment.

In commenting on these interesting findings the authors noted the
wealth of evidence for strain differences in the correlation between brain
biochemistry and behavior and pointed to some of the perplexities their
results raise in comparison, for example, with the data noted above, which
are indicative of differences which point to higher, rather than lower, brain
serotonin levels in rats of Eriksson's high-preference (AA) selected strain,
as compared with the low-preference one, the ANA (Ahtee and Eriksson,
1972, 1973; see Chapter 3). Clearly, this line of inquiry is reaching a stage at
which further advances may be imminent, despite the exacting nature of the
techniques employed. Methods for the crossbreeding of strains that differ
so markedly in their alcohol preference responses to manipulation of brain
amine levels, either centrally or peripherally, could have an important contribution to make in this connection.

The response of the C57BL/6 strain of mice to olfactory bulbectomy
was found by Nachman *et al.* (1971) to be minimal in altering their high
preference as compared with that of the BALB/c mice, who, normally aversive, were rendered much less so by surgery. The involvement of olfactory
and orosensory factors in the discriminatory mechanisms implied by these
findings was strengthened by further experimentation in which aversion to
sucrose, saccharin, and alcohol solutions was successfully conditioned in
the BALB mice, but not in the C57BL ones, by injection of lithium
chloride immediately after ingestion. The findings point rather strongly to

the latter being insensitive to the sensory cues, such as odor, which normally make alcohol aversive to the BALB mice, a conclusion reinforced by the briefly reported data of Belknap (1977). He showed that C57BL mice achieved blood alcohol concentrations twice as high as those of DBA mice—a nonpreferring strain—within 15 min of exposure to a two-bottle preference situation.

Another form of genotype–environment interaction employing the high- and low-preference strains, C57BL and DBA, was demonstrated by Randall and Lester (1975*c*), whose data suggest that caging weanling mice with a same-sex adult of the opposite preference strain under preference conditions until 10 weeks of age had a profound effect on their 10% (wt./vol.) alcohol intake scores in subsequent eight-day preference tests. The low-scoring DBA mice increased their consumption considerably, though not to the levels exhibited by their high-intake C57 adult companions, while the C57 mice attained rather more closely the low levels of the DBA mice with whom they had been housed. The authors suggested that this strong environmental effect, mediated, it will be noted, through the genotype of another mouse, was best explained in terms of a modeling hypothesis. Further work on environmental determinants was pursued by Komura *et al.* (1972) who cross-fostered half litters between the two strains and allowed pups and mother (or foster mother, as the case might be) free access to 7.9% (wt./vol.) ethanol or water. This cross-fostering procedure is the standard one for testing postnatal maternal environmental effects and in this case provided some evidence that the high preference of the C57 foster mothers affected the pups they reared, irrespective of the strain of their biological mothers, though the (opposite) effect was less marked with low-preference DBA foster mothers. Thus C57 pups drank more alcohol irrespective of the kind of rearing. Despite the authors' arguments, it would seem that the possibility cannot be excluded that the experience of imbibing alcohol in the foster mother's milk had a decisive effect in establishing alcohol preference. The reality of such a possibility was reinforced by Abel's demonstration (1975) that ethanol given to lactating rat mothers can influence the nonpreference behavior of their offspring. He showed that it increased the juveniles' open-field ambulation scores as compared with untreated controls, though among females only. Also, Ginsburg *et al.* (1977) briefly reported similar effects in C57BL and DBA mice, this time relating to both increased audiogenic seizure susceptibility and decreased aggressiveness, with DBA mice being the more affected.

Randall and Lester's (1975*b*) study of maternal influences on alcohol preference in the mouse, also using the C57BL and DBA mouse strains, suffered from the same difficulty of interpretation, though some attempt was made to evaluate the possibility by observations that the amount of alcohol consumed during the period of lactation, even by the high-preference C57 mice, was relatively small. Mice of the other, DBA, strain fostered to such mothers drank significantly more of a 7.5% (wt./vol.) ethanol solution when exposed to a choice between it and water for 7 days after weaning. The reverse fostering, that is, C57 pups reared by DBA mothers, showed no such tendency, in this case to *decrease* preference and consumption measures, as compared in each case with nonfostered control mice. But the possibility of contamination of these data by the experience by the pups themselves of the opportunity afforded them, before weaning at 25 days of age, of drinking from the tube containing alcohol, which was offered to each mother apparently at the time of parturition and thereafter, remains a real one. In this way, the C57 pups could have established their characteristic preference before the postweaning test period, irrespective of the type of mothering received, and the DBA mice reared by C57 mothers might have developed the minor though probably significant preference revealed in Randall and Lester's data by some degree of "forced" exposure via the mother's milk, confirmed later by individual experience of the aqueous solution of alcohol. This account is necessarily speculative, but it does point up the difficulties entrained by the procedure used.

The useful but not strictly necessary control for the fostering process as such was accomplished in a second experiment by transferring pups to foster mothers of the same, rather than the opposite, strain. The identity of individuals, which it is obviously of paramount importance to preserve in this manipulation, was retained by injecting a dye into a foot pad of each mouse so transferred. These preference data showed no effect of this fostering procedure when the appropriate comparisons were made, but did reveal a disturbing discrepancy between the absolute levels of the measures taken in the two experiments, which, while not calling into question the strain difference in preference as such, did suggest that its measurement is not as robust as could be wished. These differences were not, however, evaluated statistically.

The authors regard these data as confirming the findings of Komura *et al.* discussed above in that the suggestion of a maternal effect exerted by the mothers of the C57 strain is supported. As noted, there are difficulties associated with this explanation, but if we disregard them, the next step in the way in which an analysis of such an effect might proceed is to attempt to discover when the effect is mediated, either prenatally or postnatally. The point here is that even if present postnatally, its origin may be traceable to the influence of the mother on the development of her offspring *in utero*, which, of course, is not controlled for by the cross-fostering procedure alone. The necessary control for prenatal environmental effects is achieved by reciprocal crossing of strains. In the event that the strains are inbred, that is genetically homozygous at least at the loci governing the phenotype in question as is presumably the case with the C57 and DBA mice currently under discussion, the F_1 cross is naturally heterozygous at all these loci. But it is uniformly heterozygous, and hence it should be a matter of indifference which strain is used as the mother and which as the father. Thus, the reciprocal crosses should, within the limits of error, be identical. If they are not and display a resemblance to the female parent, then a *prima facie* case for a prenatal maternal effect can be presumed, and the causes of it may be investigated further. Two possible candidates can be considered. First, if sex linkage is operating, then it will show itself as a difference between the two F_1s—in one of them, only the female offspring would resemble the mothers, the males being like the fathers. Second, if the cause is cytoplasmic inheritance—that is, an effect due to extranuclear nonchromosomal material, which is more abundantly contributed to the zygote on fertilization by the larger amount of such material contributed by the female gamete, the ovum, than by the smaller-sized male spermatozoon—then an appropriate technique for its analysis is the transplantation of such fertilized ova into the uterus of recipients of the two opposing strains. A positive finding, that is, a maternal effect despite such cross-strain transfers would point to extranuclear inheritance, whereas a negative one would imply that the effect was attributable to the uterine environment peculiar to one strain. Broadhurst (1961) gave the outline of a scheme for the analysis of behavioral phenotypes for which a maternal effect is suspected, which incorporates these possibilities and which is reproduced as Table XIV.

Randall and Lester (1975*a*) omit reciprocal crossing, however, and proceed directly to ova transplantation. There are, nevertheless, data that bear on the analysis of prenatal effects on alcohol preference as may be derived from the reciprocal crossings reported in the literature, none of which indicate maternal effects involving the C57 strain. An early example was supplied by McClearn and Rodgers (1961) who were unable to find any significant difference between reciprocal crosses of the C57BL and C3H strains. Thus the status of the investigation of Randall and Lester is ambiguous, since what is under test in an investigation involving ova transplantation is not the existence of a maternal effect, but its causation. The claim that the technique can, in and of itself, unravel the complexities of the genetic and environmental determinants of behavior is unfounded. Moreover, the work reported is open to several objections. First, if the offspring, both those derived from ova recovered after fertilization and transferred to one uterine horn of a pregnant female of the opposite strain, and those nurtured *in utero* in the normal way, were raised by mothers having access to alcohol, as in their previous experiment—and their report is unclear on this point—then the same objections remain. Second, control transplants were

TABLE XIV

Scheme to Show Possible Matings Between Two Strains, High (H) and Low (L),
Needed to Display Any Maternal Effects[a]

| Type of effect | Type of treatment | Type of mating | | Prenatal environment (uterine) | Postnatal environment (to weaning) |
		Female	Male		
I. Postnatal	Cross-fostering[b]	H ×	H	H	L
		H ×	H	H	H
		L ×	L	L	H
		L ×	L	L	L
II. Prenatal	A. Reciprocal crosses[c]	H ×	L	H	H
		L ×	H	L	L
	B. Transplanted ova[b,c]	H ×	H	L	L
		H ×	H	H	H
		L ×	L	H	H
		L ×	L	L	L

[a]Reproduced from Broadhurst (1961).
[b]In I and IIB the normal procedure with which each experimental treatment is to be compared is shown on the line below.
[c]In IIA and B the possible further variations between pre- and postnatal maternal environment, as given in I, are not shown.

undertaken, that is, within strain, to assess the effect on the postweaning 7-day preference test in the way used before of the transplantation pro cedure as such, independently of strain. But the identity of the transplanted subjects was lost, since they could not be identified by the coat- and eye-color differences—C57BL mice being black and the DBA mice dilute brown—in the way used to separate transplanted pups from non-transplanted ones in the mixed-strain litters derived from the cross-strain transfers. This point is especially important since litters were culled to four at birth. The analyses presented do not separate these within-strain transfers from a further control group of mice reared without any experimental intervention. Nor is it clear if the nontransferred offspring of the mothers, which served as recipients for the cross-strain transplants—another obvious control for comparison—were included in the analyses. These methodological problems, which, together with others, have been pointed out by Joffe *et al.* (1976), render Randall and Lester's conclusion that their results ". . . support the genetic basis of alcohol selection in the C57BL mouse, . . . while demonstrating that alcohol avoidance in DBA mice is subject to environmental manipulation" (pp. 147–148) so fraught with uncertainties, to say nothing of the rigidity of the dichotomy implied in the terms in which it is couched, as to be almost meaningless as a statement about genotype–environment interaction on alcohol preference.

Yet another interaction of strain with environmental variables has been reported by Goodrick (1972) in a methodological contribution bearing on the preference measurement. A preference for drinking tap water from the end bottles when confronted with an array of five or seven spouts appeared to interact with strain (and sex) among three mouse strains, including the C57BL/6J. But the possibility of artifacts arising from social interaction, for example, territorial, between the rather large numbers of individuals (6–8) caged together makes the bearing these findings might have on the ethanol preference data presented somewhat speculative.

Schneider *et al.* (1973) confirmed once again the established ethanol preference of the C57BL strain in comparisons with others and in relation to effects of forced alcohol consumption in disrupting nest building as a measure of behavioral competence, and of injection of alcohol in suppressing the jaw-jerk reflex response to faradic stimulation as a measure of neural competence. The C57BL/6J were more resisitant to both than the two low-preference strains used (DBA/2J and Swiss–Webster). Ethanol metabolism was also confirmed as relatively similar in the C57BL and DBA strains, but an ingenious attempt to test the hypothesis that postingestional effects were important in preference determination by offering a choice between water and an alcohol, 1,2-propanediol (propylene glycol), which does not metabolize to the toxic acetaldehyde as does ethanol, failed to yield the increase in preference by the DBA strain that the hypothesis would lead one to expect. This finding, it should be noted, is in some opposition to Sheppard *et al.* (1970) who showed rather clearly that the DBA strain shows a biochemically significant lower level of aldehyde dehydrogenase in the blood than the C57 mice, which allows the DBA strain an increased accumulation of acetaldehyde after ethanol injection to an extent that could account for their behavioral aversion. Dudek (1977) sought to test this proposition directly by establishing a taste aversion (to saccharin) reinforced by injections of acetaldehyde, which was then measured in later preference tests. The DBA mice showed the most pronounced aversion, and F_1 cross between them and C57 mice was intermediate and the C57BL parental strain was least affected by the acetaldehyde. But sleep times in response to the drug reversed the strains with the hybrids showing potence for long times, like the C57 mice. The findings of Belknap *et al.* (1972), on the other hand, point away from any difference between the C57BL/6J strain they used and the DBA/2J (as well as the BALB/cJ) with respect to their aldehyde dehydrogenase observed at a range of times after a single injection of 3.55 g/kg of ethanol. The ethanol-induced sleep time (see Chapter 3) in response to this dose was markedly shorter in the C57 group, which showed a significant increase in alcohol dehydrogenase as compared to controls drawn from the same strains. Coupled with evidence of some degree of correlation (-0.57) between sleep time and alcohol dehydrogenase activity, derived, however, from McClearn's heterozygous mouse strain (HS, see Section 7.3), these results point to the importance of hepatic metabolism variables.

But variations in neural sensitivity between C57 mice and other mouse strains remain the most favored explanation of Schneider *et al.*, and they suggest that differences—possibly morphological, possibly biochemical—in neural membranes may underlie the genotype–environment interaction so frequently demonstrated with these phenotypes. In further work, Schneider *et al.* (1974) extended the finding regarding the unusual resistance of the C57BL/6J strain to the suppression of the jaw-jerk reflex after ethanol by showing that yet another strain, the BALB/cJ, did not share it. Hillman and Schneider (1975) confirmed the finding of the greater preference of C57BL strain mice for propanediol, in contrast, in this case, to that of no less than three other strains, including the DBA, which shows low preference for this alcohol. Injecting 5.0 ml/kg of propanediol increased the open-field activity of the C57 mice 15, 30, and 45 min afterward, whereas only the CBA among the other strains gave evidence of an increase and that at the 45-min postinjection interval only. Sleep times after ethanol gave congruent results so that the similarity of the strain-dependent behavioral effects of the two alcohols appears well established. Strange *et al.* (1976) continued this approach, using three further alcohols. Among them l-propanol yielded the same preference differential in favor of the C57 strain, which was also more resistant to the effects of injections of the drugs with respect to open-field test activity scores. McClearn and Shern (1975) briefly indicated that five strains' responses to injected ethanol in open-field ambulation scores showed an interaction with dose, and Randall *et al.* (1975) reported that C57BL and BALB mice responded differently to increasing doses of ethanol (0.75, 1.50, and 2.25 g/kg, i.p.). The activity of C57 mice, as measured in stabilimeter cages, decreased with dose, whereas that of the BALB strain remained the same or increased slightly. The latter finding, though not the former, is at variance with data on the same strain in Oliverio and Eleftheriou's somewhat larger study of the same phenotype (1976—see Chapter 8).

Isolation as an experiential variable can also affect the relative standing of mouse strains. Yanai and Ginsburg (1976) reported an interaction between strain (C57BL/10 and DBA/1) and treatment (isolation versus groupings of six mice) in the number of days to survival after imposition of a liquid diet containing 4.7% (wt./vol.) ethanol. The C57 mice proved to be significantly more robust overall, as did the grouped mice, compared with those that had been fed ethanol in isolation, though the deleterious effects of isolation were not uniformly significant at both of the two ages (36 and 50 days) studied. The significantly greater alcohol intake of isolated mice, possibly a function of a reduced plasma corticosterone level, was doubtless the most important factor in determining this drug–strain interaction.

The work of Damjanovich and MacInnes (1973; MacInnes and Damjanovich, 1973) would seem to add further support to the special status of the C57BL strain. Their analyses of responses to injected ethanol in three of the strains previously discussed (C57BL/6J, DBA/2J, and BALB/c), again using ethanol-induced sleep times, now coupled with fall times (the length of time the mouse could continue clinging to a wire screen) as well as blood-alcohol assays, showed that the C57 strain's greater resistance to the effects of alcohol, as seen in their shorter sleep times and longer fall times over a range of dose levels as compared with the other two strains, lies in blood-alcohol clearance rate, which they monitored by blood assays. This measure showed a drug–strain interaction, itself modified by dosage of the ethanol used to challenge the genotype, but not unequivocally establishing the superiority of the C57 mice in resisting the challenge at all the dose levels used. Damjanovich and MacInnes (1973) presented a useful tabulation of the various findings of McClearn's group on the standing of the three strains, C57BL, DBA, and BALB, in measures of sensitivity to ethanol, which is reproduced as Table XV.

Randall and Lester (1974) added a further dimension to the discussion

TABLE XV

Comparisons of Effects of, or Reactions to, Ethanol Challenge in Mice of Three Inbred Strains[a]

Reference	Parameter	C57BL/6J	DBA/2J	BALB/cJ
Rodgers and McClearn (1962b)	Alcohol drinking preference	High[b]	Very low[b]	Intermediate[b]
Damjanovich and MacInnes (1973)	Sleep time (at high dose)	Low[b,c]	High[b]	High[c]
Belknap et al. (1973)	Alcohol dehydrogenase activity	High[b]	Low[b,c]	High[c]
Belknap et al. (1973)	Aldehyde dehydrogenase activity	Moderate[b]	Moderate[c]	Low[b,c]
MacInnes and Uphouse (1973)	Interference with task acquisition	Low[b]	High[b]	—
MacInnes and Uphouse (1973)	Effects on exploration of novel situation	Decrease[b]	Increase[b]	—
Damjanovich and MacInnes (1973)	Tissue sensitivity, by "minimum narcotic dose" method	Intermediate	Low	High
Damjanovich and MacInnes (1973)	Tissue sensitivity, by waking blood alcohol level	Intermediate[b]	Low[b]	High[b]
Damjanovich and MacInnes (1973)	Tissue sensitivity, by blood alcohol level at unconsciousness	Intermediate[b]	Low[b]	High[b]

[a]From Damjanovich and MacInnes (1973).
[b,c]Indicate significant differences ($p < .05$) for between-strain comparisons at that parameter. Comparisons are between strains with like symbols [letters].

by comparing C57BL/6J and BALB/cJ strains with respect not only to their difference in sleep time after ethanol (confirming the previously reported resistance of the former), but also of their sleep after pentobarbital. Injection of 50 mg/kg revealed no significant difference between them in sleep times, but there was some indication that the C57 mice metabolized the drug faster, pointing to a greater neural sensitivity on their part. Be that as it may, these findings suggest that the drug–strain interaction in response to injected ethanol usually encountered in comparisons involving the C57BL strain may be one that is specific to alcohols. Neither is this interaction absolute, in that it can be abolished, as Ho *et al.* (1975) have demonstrated. They used a choline acetyltransferase, 4-(1-naphthylvinyl) pyridium salt (NVP), a 10-mg/kg injection of which served to reduce temporarily the preference for a 3.9% (wt./vol.) solution of ethanol, so that equal amounts of the solution and water were drunk. These authors also concerned themselves with the observed level of various neurotransmitters in whole-brain homogenates of the two strains used. The C57BL/6J mice exceeded the DBA/2J mice only with respect to acetylcholine, with the DBA being higher in acetylcholinesterase, levels of norepinephrine, dopamine, and serotonin being nonsignificantly different from each other. The absence of differences in brain serotonin between the same two strains was confirmed by Pickett and Collins (1975), who nevertheless proceeded to attempt a genetic analysis by crossbreeding to produce F_1 and F_2 filial crosses, though not backcrosses, the rationale advanced being that information about genetic correlation between this phenotype and that of preference behavior might assist in resolving the ambiguities in the literature about the possible causal relation between them. Such a limited breeding design can hardly be expected to resolve such a question, especially when appropriate analysis for quantitative variation was not applied and genetic variation in brain serotonin is not indicated by any of the generational values. On the other hand, the difference in preference between the subline used (C57BL/Ibg) and DBA/2 (subline not stated) was yet again confirmed, and the data presented did show the absence of reciprocal differences (indicative of no prenatal maternal effects) and the existence of some directional dominance in favor of low preference. Yet another neurotransmitter, γ-aminobutyric acid (GABA), has been eliminated as a variable by Chan (1976) who also studied its regional distribution in the brains of male mice of the same C57BL/6J and DBA/2J strains at various intervals after a single injection of 4 mg/kg of ethanol, the time range now being extended to include values up to 170 min after injection. As with comparable work on the LS and SS selected strains (see Chapter 3), the dosage used raised GABA levels over saline controls, generally significantly, especially in the thalamus–hypothalamus region, but strain differences were absent.

The nature of the individuality of the C57 mice in ethanol sensitivity has been further examined by Goldstein and Kakihana (1974) who used the former's technique (Goldstein, 1973) of fuming combined with pyrazole injections (see Chapter 3) to demonstrate that the C57BL/6J strain's relative resistance to the subsequent seizures on withdrawl from alcohol treatment paralleled their similar response to reserpine-induced convulsions compared, in both cases, with mice of the DBA and Swiss–Webster strains. Previous forced intake of alcohol over a prolonged period (up to 20 weeks) did not greatly affect the outcome, though there was some evidence of a drug–strain interaction with respect to this treatment. The pretreated C57 mice showed a consistently lower blood-alcohol level during the three days' fuming than did the pretreated DBA mice as compared with their non-pretreated controls in each case, as well as an overall lower level, reflecting their greater resistance to alcohol. The difference was, however, insufficient to account for the marked difference in their seizure susceptibility referred to above. Possible explanatory mechanisms depending on differences in physical dependence, in sensitivity of the central nervous system, and in brain biochemistry were discussed. The role of acetaldehyde (see earlier) in mediating withdrawal symptoms was noted by Thurman and Pathman (1975) as equivocal, since the C57BL strain, which had the slightly higher blood levels of acetaldehyde following exposure to ethanol and antabuse, displayed much less intense withdrawal reactions than the DBA mice.

The effect of major coat-color genes on alcohol preference in the mouse has been reported by Henry and Schlesinger (1967) in the context of a study of several behavioral phenotypes, including avoidance conditioning and audiogenic seizure susceptibility. They used stocks of C57BL/6J mice among which, as a result of previous crossbreeding with an albino strain, segregation for albinism was occurring; that is, some individuals were homozygous albino, whereas their litter mates were either heterozygous, and hence colored (black) since the albino allele is recessive, or homozygous for black. The black mice as a group had significantly higher preference ratios for 7.9% (wt./vol.) ethanol than the white. The value of this observation was lessened by the lack of intake measures and by the absence of an evaluation of the effects of a single dose of the albino gene, concealed among the black group. To reveal its effects, progeny testing of these colored subjects would have been necessary. A parallel study of the dilute locus (*d*—see Section 7.3) on a DBA/2J background showed no significant effect on preference ratios.

This finding was confirmed by Fuller and Collins (1972) both for the dilute locus and for another locus, *b*, concerned with coat color in the mouse, in a study that nevertheless presented an analysis of the genetics of preference using the same two strains just referred to above. Data from a complete Mendelian cross, that is, parental strains and both filial crosses and backcrosses, were collected and analyzed according to a nonparametric method not yet sufficiently well described in the literature to enable evaluation of it. Nevertheless a good fit with a two-factor model—where the "factors" could be major genes or linked groups of genes akin to Mather and Jinks' (1971) "effective factors"—was claimed. The need is obvious for confirmation of this interesting suggestion by further analysis, for which the approach using recombinant and congenic strains (see Chapter 8) might perhaps be appropriate.

Further work on the possible modification of the effects of alcohol by albinism is briefly reported by Rush and King (1976), who used comparable C57 material to study their alcohol sleep times. Black genotypes were less sensitive on this measure than were the albino. Various other crosses were generated to insure the segregation of the albino locus against a uniform genotypic background: In all cases the albinos slept longer than the pigmented stocks, though not always significantly so among females.

The direct effects of ethanol on other learned behaviors of rodents continue to be studied. Baum (1971) showed that two strains of mice not among those referred to above, the AKR and the A/Jax, did not differ significantly with respect to the number of active avoidance responses made during an extinction session following intraperitoneal injection of alcohol, though there was some suggestion of a differential effect due to strain at the higher (1.184 g/kg) of the two doses used. MacInnes and Uphouse (1973) similarly studied acquisition as well as extinction not of active, but of passive, avoidance, though reverting to the more familiar C57BL/6 and DBA/2 strains. In addition, an F_1 cross was made, but not reciprocally, and these subjects were included in the range—0.5–3.0 g/kg—of doses injected intraperitoneally 15–20 min before the first day of training. Mice were required to remain in the start compartment as opposed to moving into another, black one, in which they received foot shock, and on the second day, on which no shock was given, retention of the passive-avoidance response was measured. All groups showed some impairment of acquisition, as compared with saline controls, though this impairment was probably not statistically significant until the higher doses were reached. However, the C57 mice were less affected than the DBA, and the F_1 between them tended to resemble the former rather than the latter; that is, there was potence for poor acquisition under the effects of alcohol. The retention data showed some evidence for state dependence of recall of the initial response tested over a more limited dose range, in that latencies for moving from the starting compartment were depressed when tested under saline after acquisition under ethanol, as compared with saline–saline groups, depressed latency scores here, of course, being indicative of poorer retention of the avoidance response. But these effects were not uniform across the genetic groupings, the F_1 in particular showing little evidence of state dependence; indeed, they showed some heterotic effects in that on retesting under saline after acquisition under alcohol, their scores at the 1.5- and 2.0-g/kg doses transcended those of the two parental strains, which showed considerably poorer retention. The authors invoked genetic buffering (Fulker, 1970) as an explanation, but the problems associated with explanations of this kind based merely on phenotypic resemblances (see Chapter 6) make such suggestions, interesting though they may be, inevitably speculative without the support a more extensive examination of the genetic architecture could yield.

Strain differences between the C57 black and DBA mice with respect to aggressive behavior were studied by Yanai *et al.* (1976) using the previously reported technique (see Section 7.3) of forcing ingestion of 7.9% alcohol for prolonged periods, including pregnancy and parturition. The offspring of the normally more aggressive DBA/1/Bg mice showed considerable reduction in indices of fighting; the less aggressive C57BL/10/Bg animals showed a similar but smaller reduction, which suggests that this interesting drug–strain interaction may be a scalar artifact resulting from a "floor" effect of the kind suspected in some of Buxton's (1974) work (Chapter 4).

Further attempts to establish the genetic architecture of preference in rats and mice have been reported since the major reviews referred to above, though an early attempt by Thomas (1969) does not seem to have attracted attention, perhaps because of a certain indeterminacy in the techniques of preference measurement employed. While she used a classical Mendelian pattern of crossing parental mouse strains—the C57BL/Crgl and the DBA/Crgl—to breed their first and second filial crosses, together with backcrosses, numbers in some of the derived generations were very small (as few as five), and reliance was placed on threshold responses to concentrations as low as 0.01% ethanol. It is not surprising that scaling difficulties were reported as preventing any appropriate analysis of the data.

In contrast, Whitney *et al.* (1970) reviewed previous progress in establishing heritability estimates using both inbred and selectively bred strains and theirs is probably the most sophisticated analysis of data on the heritability of alcohol preference using methods of quantitative genetics. Their treatment subsumes Brewster's reanalyses (1968) of the previous mouse data of McClearn and Rodgers (1961), who used the classical parental, filial, and backcross generations, and of those of Fuller (1964), who used, as was noted later (Fuller and Collins, 1972), a breeding pattern that constituted a half-diallel cross of four inbred strains of mice, and included a commentary on Brewster's (1968, 1972) own diallel analysis of preference among rat strains derived from selection (see Chapter 4). In addition, they presented new data of their own on the mouse, using both the classical method mentioned above and techniques of parent–offspring and sibling correlation, including some values from the S_{10} generation of the bidirectional selection in the mouse for extremes of activity in the open field (DeFries and Hegmann, 1970) mentioned in Chapter 4. The estimates they derived, in contrast to those of Brewster, were all rather low and of the order of 40% or less. Some of the reasons for the differences, which they explored, were essentially technical ones and related to the formulas used, but they were impressed by the degree of uniformity that they had been able to detect both across species (rat and mouse) and across the diverse methodologies used. This uniformity led Whitney *et al.* to question the conventional wisdom current in psychogenetics, which insists that heritabilities are a population parameter and hence not to be generalized across populations, let alone species, and to suggest that the heritability of a character may not be specific to a particular population. But if variation in alcohol preference can be shown to depend on a relatively simple physiological mechanism common to all rodents—or, at least, to rats and mice, and one which, even if it proves not to be simple physiologically, has a pattern of genetic determination which is similar in kind and comparable in terms of gene action—then, of course, both views may be tenable. On the other hand, it may be that the congruence in the figures, which Whitney *et al.* perceive, is fortuitous, albeit impressive. This latter possibility is rendered less likely by Reed's briefly reported study (1976) of responses in McClearn's HS mice to ethanol as measured in a variety of behaviors (not, however, including preference). Parent–offspring heritabilities, where significantly different from zero, were all rather low, 0.21 (for sleep time) being the highest.

Whitney's further contribution (1972) to the analysis of genetic architecture of the preference phenotype consisted of a multivariate genotype–environment study in which an environmental dimension was deliberately introduced into the design. This can be an especially powerful approach when associated with a breeding study of adequate proportions (Broadhurst *et al.*, 1974). As in several other examples now extant in the psychogenetical literature, the aspect of the macroenvironment manipulated was not the ingestion of a pharmacological agent, in the manner the reader will have become familiar with in many experiments reviewed in this book, but the imposition of stress in the adult. This procedure consisted of exposing the subjects of the first and second filial generations, bred from a cross between the high-preference C57BL mice and the JK/Bi, a low-preference strain, to naturalistic stress of a kind designed to heighten alarm. This stress was the playing at loud volume of the cries of mice receiving strong electric shock, which was relayed to subjects during, first, a preference test for 7.9% ethanol lasting 14 days, then an open-field test and, finally, an emergence test. While the stressor resulted in lowered values for preference (and increased emotional indices) in both inbred strains, it affected the derived generations but little, in a manner reminiscent of "buffering," or resistance to environmental displacement of the phenotype in hybrid material, though Whitney did not pursue this aspect of the analysis to the extent of being able to specify the origin of the determination of such buffering as was shown, for example, in Fulker's (1970) specification of maternal involvement in the determination of hybrids' resistance to stress. Instead he concentrated on analyses that provided the basis for genetic correlation between some of the various phenotypes measured. The values for preference and open-field defecation (-0.68) and preference and open-field urination (-0.81) reflect the extent to which there is a commonality in the additive component of the genetic determination of the phenotypes in question and, though probably imprecise, are quite large despite the low *phenotypic* correlations reported between the variables in question and the even lower correlations based on the environmental components of the variation observed. However, it is not clear from the published report whether or not the variation due to the stress imposed was included in the analysis, so that the power of the method may not have been fully exploited in this case.

Eriksson (1971*a*) attempted a similar analysis with perhaps even less success: He used taste preference as the macroenvironmental manipulation similar to that used in his selection experiment (see Chapter 3), namely, the addition of saccharin to the alcohol solution and quinine to the water. He also used the high-preference C57BL mice, but the low-preference behavior was supplied by the CBA/Ca strain. The classical Mendelian crossing design was completed by breeding backcrosses to the parental strains from the first (F_1) of the two filial generations, and all subjects were tested under both normal and manipulated-choice conditions. The effect of the latter was to increase the intake of alcohol in all groups, though one, the females of the C57BL parental strain, was already ingesting as much alcohol as it was able to metabolize, and hence this group increased its scores very little. These artifacts in part occasioned scaling problems not altogether resolved by various transformations. Such can be applied to psychogenetic data for the purpose of retaining simple biometrical models in order to avoid adding parameters that complicate the genetical models used, but which may become necessary to accomplish a satisfactory analysis of the data (Jinks and Broadhurst, 1974). It cannot, however, be said that the analyses reported are at all satisfactory, and in particular the reliance on the simple (and outmoded) methods of Bruell (1962) for the estimation of the degree of dominance variation is unfortunate. While there is no doubt of the fact of potence (phenotypic dominance) for low preference under both environmental conditions in Eriksson's data, once again it must be said that the pitfalls inherent in regarding the location of the F_1 on a metrical scale as a guide to the direction of expression in their action on the phenotype of dominance components of variation, in the way briefly explored in relation to Anisman's work (see Chapter 6), have not been demonstrably avoided. However, the mean values reported for the backcross generations supported the interpretation of directional dominance for low preference. This finding is in some opposition to that of Brewster's reanalysis (1968) of Fuller's half-diallel cross (1964) of four strains including the C57BL but not the CBA, mentioned above in connection with the work of Whitney *et al.* (1970). Brewster showed rather convincingly that there was some association between the moderate degree of genetic dominance displayed by Fuller's four strains and the extent of their phenotypic preference for alcohol; that is to say, there was dominance for *high* preference. Moreover, the C57BL strain was shown, by the covariance–variance graph technique, to be the strain with the largest proportion of dominant to recessive genes in its makeup. Further work is obviously needed to encompass this apparent discrepancy, and the heritabilities reported by Eriksson bear little on it. Calculated by methods that seem generally appropriate, they ranged in the region of 35%, that is, toward the upper limit of those discussed by Whitney *et al.* (1970). Of perhaps greater interest than the actual values is the fact that they do not differ much as between the two conditions of preference testing, so that there is no evidence of genotype–environment interaction involving this pharmacological phenotype and its distortion by taste preferences in the strains of mouse studied.

This concludes our review of more recent work on the genetics of alcohol preference and response to alcohol in animals, subsequent to that cited at the beginning of this chapter. A summary of the findings will be found in Table XVI.

9.2. Opiates and Barbiturates

As was the case with our survey of work on the pharmacogenetics of alcohol preference studied by methods of selection (Chapter 3), we encounter considerably less research on other drugs of dependence, especially morphine, studied in this case by methods of strain differences and crossbreeding. Reports of differences between strains of mice, not ones we have come to recognize as rather standard ones in psychogenetics, are noted, for example, by Way *et al.* (1969) and Brase *et al.* (1974). In both cases they are only incidental to the main themes of research, but indicate

TABLE XVI

Recent Psychopharmacogenetic Experiments with Alcohol

Reference	Species (and strain)	Treatment	Measure	Outcome	Remarks
Poley and Mos (1974)	Mouse, SWR/J/ SJL/J, and deer mice		Behavior battery, ethanol preference	Correlation between emotionality and preference	Confirms Poley *et al.* (1970)
Kahn (1974)	Mouse, C3H/AEj, CFI		Alcohol preference	Both strains averse, especially young adults	
Poley(1972)	Mouse, C57BL/6A		Ethanol preference	No preference shown	Atypical for C57
Wise (1974)	Rat, Wistar, Sprague–Dawley		Alcohol preference	Instability of strain differences	Genetic drift?
Anisman and Waller (1974)	Rat, Sprague–Dawley Holtzman		Alcohol preference after shock	No strain difference	Male rats only
Melchior and Myers (1976)	Rat, Sprague–Dawley Holtzman, Long–Evans, Wistar	5,6-DHT, 6-OHDA, 5,7-DHT (not Long–Evans), intra-cerebral injection	Alcohol preference before treatment, 10 and 60 days after	Drug-strain interactions 5,6-DHT increased all but Wistar 6-OHDA decreased all but Holtzman 5,7-DHT no effect	
Nachman *et al.* (1971)	Mouse, C57BL/6, BALB/c	Olfactory bulbectomy	Alcohol preference	C57 unchanged BALB reduced aversion	
		Lithium chloride after sucrose, saccharin, and alcohol ingestion	Alcohol preference	BALB made aversive but not C57	BALB sensitive to aversive odor of alcohol (Belknap, 1977)
Randall and Lester (1975c)	Mouse, C57BL, DBA	Caged weanling mice with same-sex adult of opposite prefer-ence strain until 10 weeks	Alcohol preference	DBA decreased aversion C57 decreased preference	Modeling?
Komura *et al.* (1972)	Mouse, C57BL, DBA	Cross-fostered	Ethanol preference	Pups reared by C57 mothers increased preference. No change when reared by DBA mothers	Does alcohol in milk affect preference?

Reference	Subjects	Treatment	Behavior measured	Results	Comments
Thomas (1969)	Mouse, C57BL/Crgl, DBA/2Crgl, and F_1, F_2, backcross		Alcohol preference	Preference related to proportion of C57 genes in a group	Scaling difficulties
Whitney et al. (1970)	Mouse, C57BL/1Bi, JK/Bi, C57BL/Crgl, DBA/2Crgl, and Mendelian cross		Heritability of ethanol preference	Heritability = 0.10–0.15	May be less population specific than generally supposed
Reed (1976)	Mouse, HS	Alcohol	Battery of tests	Heritability = 0.12–0.21 for open field, heart rate, and sleep time	
Whitney (1972)	Mouse, C57BL, JK/Bi, F_1, F_2	Stress	Alcohol preference, open-field emergence test	Lowered preference in P_1, P_2, but not F_1, F_2 Correlation between preference and open field, defecation, and urination	Buffering?
Eriksson (1971a)	Mouse, C57BL, CBA, and Mendelian cross		Alcohol preference under normal and taste-preference conditions	Taste preference increased in all groups Heritability of 35% under both conditions	Scaling problems Directional dominance for low preference? Opposes Brewster (1968)
Amit et al. (1976)	Rat, Sprague–Dawley, Wistar	Injections of disulfiram, FLA-63, or calcium carbamide	Ethanol preference blood acetaldehyde level	No strain difference	Disulfiram acts against alcohol by inhibition of dopamine-beta-hydroxylase
Yanai and Ginsburg (1976)	Mouse, C57BL/10, DBA/1	Isolation vs. groups	Days to survival after ethanol-rich liquid diet	Isolation-strain interaction. C57's and grouped mice more robust	
Randall et al. (1975)	Mouse, C57BL, BALB	Ethanol, range of doses	Activity in stabilimeter cages	C57 decreased with dose. BALB same or increased slightly with dose	Opposes Oliverio and Eleftheriou (1976)

(Continued)

TABLE XVI—*Continued*

Reference	Species (and strain)	Treatment	Measure	Outcome	Remarks
Damjanovich and MacInnes (1973) MacInnes and Damjanovich (1973)	Mouse, C57BL/6J, DBA/2J, BALB/c	Ethanol, range of doses	Sleep times, fall times, and blood alcohol assays	C57 shortest sleep times, longest fall times. Assay showed drug-strain interaction	
Randall and Lester (1974)	Mouse, C57BL/6J, BALB/cJ	Ethanol Pentobarbital	Sleep time	C57 greatest resistance No significant difference	C57 greater neural sensitivity?
Ho et al. (1975)	Mouse, C57BL/6J, DBA/2J	NVP to reduce ethanol preference	Levels of neuro-transmitters	C57 higher in acetylcholine. DBA higher in acetyl-cholinesterase	
Pickett and Collins (1975)	Mouse, C57BL/1bg, DBA/2, F_1 and F_2		Alcohol preference Measure of brain serotonin levels	C57 greatest preference No significant difference	Attempted genetic analysis
Goldstein and Kakihana (1974)	Mouse, C57BL/6J, DBA, Swiss Webster	Fuming combined with pyrazole injections Ethanol then fuming combined with pyrazole injections	Seizure suscept-ibility after alcohol withdrawal Seizure suscept-ibility after alcohol withdrawal	C57 most resistant C57 most resistant	C57 lowest blood alcohol level during fuming
Chan (1976)	Mouse, C57BL/6J, DBA/2J	Ethanol injection	Brain GABA content	Raised, especially in thalamus/hypo-thalamus. No strain differences	
Ginsburg et al. (1977)	Mouse, C57BL, DBA	Ethanol given to lactating mothers	Audiogenic seizure susceptibility of offspring Aggression of offspring	Increased Decreased	DBAs more affected in both measures

Reference	Animal/Strain	Treatment	Measure	Result	Comments
Randall and Lester (1975b)	Mouse, C57BL, DBA	Cross-fostering between strains	Ethanol preference of offspring	DBA pups reared by C57 mothers increased preference. No change in DBA pups or any reared by DBA mothers	Preferences may have been established before. Confirms Komura et al. (1972)
		Fostering within strain	Ethanol preference of offspring	No effect	Discrepancy between measures in both experiments
Randall and Lester (1975a)	Mouse, C57BL, DBA	Ova transplantation	Ethanol preference of offspring	C57 ova in DBA uterus showed increased preference. DBA ova in C57 uterus also showed increased preference	Methodological problems
Goodrick (1972)	Mouse, C57BL/6J, A/J, C3HeB/FeJ		Positional preference for water bottle	Interaction with strain and sex	Possibility of artifacts
Schneider et al. (1973)	Mouse, C57BL/6J, DBA/2J, Swiss Webster	Ethanol	Disruption of nest building; suppression of jaw-jerk reflex	C57 more resistant in both measures	Ethanol metabolism similar in C57 and DBA
			Choice between water and propylene glycol	No increase in preference of DBA	Opposes Sheppard et al. (1970)
Dudek (1977)	Mouse, DBA/2, C57BL/6, F_1 cross	Saccharin and acetaldehyde	Saccharin preference	DBA greatest aversion; C57 least affected; DBA × C57 intermediate	
Belknap et al. (1972)	Mouse, C57BL/6J, DBA/2J, BALB/cJ		Sleep times	F_1 cross and C57 long sleep time; DBA short sleep time	
			Sleep time and hepatic ADH activity	C57 shortest sleep time and increased ADH	
Schneider et al. (1974)	Mouse, C57BL/6J, BALB/cJ	No treatment	Suppression of jaw-jerk reflex	C57 resistant, but not BALB	
Hillman and Schneider (1975)	Mouse, C57BL/6J, DBA/2J, CBA/J, BALB/cJ	Propanediol	Propanediol preference	C57 greatest preference	
			Open-field activity	Increased in C57 and CBA	
		Ethanol	Sleep times	Shortest in C57	

(Continued)

TABLE XVI—*Continued*

Reference	Species (and strain)	Treatment	Measure	Outcome	Remarks
Strange *et al.* (1976)	Mouse, C57BL/6J, DBA/2J	No treatment	*1*-Propanol preference	Greatest in C57	
		1-Propanol	Open-field activity	Increased in DBA/2J	
McClearn and Shern (1975)	Mouse, 5 strains	Ethanol, range of doses	Open-field ambulation	Interaction of strain and dose	
Thurman and Pathman (1975)	Mouse, C57BL, DBA	Ethanol and antabuse	Blood level of acetaldehyde after withdrawal of alcohol	C57 lowest levels of acetaldehyde	
Henry and Schlesinger (1967)	Mouse, C57BL/6J (albino locus mutations), DBA/2J (dilute locus mutations)		Ethanol preference	Black mice had higher preference than white	Methodological problems
Fuller and Collins (1972)	Mouse, C57BL/6J (*b*-locus coat color mutations), DBA/2J (dilute locus mutations), and Mendelian cross		Alcohol preference	No significant differences	Attempted genetic analysis—two loci involved
Rush and King (1976)	Mouse, C57BL/6J (albino locus mutations)	Alcohol	Sleep times	Albino sleep longer than pigmented	
Baum (1971)	Mouse, AKR, A/Jax	Alcohol	Number of active avoidances during extinction	No difference except at higher dose	
MacInnes and Uphouse (1973)	Mouse, C57BL/6, DBA/2, F₁ cross	Alcohol, range of doses	Number of passive avoidances	C57 less affected than DBA; F₁ resembles C57	
		Saline	Number of passive avoidances	Less affected than alcohol-treated mice	
Yanai *et al.* (1976)	Mouse, C57BL, DBA/1/Bg	Alcohol during pregnancy and parturition	Aggression	Decreased aggression, greatest in DBA	May be "floor" effect

differences between strains in the extent to which mice addicted to morphine will show hyperalgesic jumping in response to injections of naloxone. This compound is a morphine antagonist that precipitates a withdrawal reaction in morphine-dependent rats and mice.

Sinclair *et al.* (1973) showed no difference between two strains of rats (Wistar albinos and Long-Evans hooded) with respect to the extent to which they demonstrated the suppression of ethanol preference induced by a single dose of morphine, whereas Tilson and Rech (1974), using two other rat strains similarly contrasted with respect to coat color (Fischer and Sprague-Dawley albinos), found differences in some behavioral and other indices of this drug's effects, but not in others. Thus the two strains showed a similar dose-response curve to the analgesic effects of morphine as measured by the threshold of flinching in response to shock, but a drug-strain interaction in that the Sprague-Dawley rats had significantly elevated thresholds after treatment with morphine. It was this strain that was most affected by pretreatment with *p*-chlorophenylalanine, a serotonin depletor (see Chapter 3), in that 97 hr after the start of daily injections of the inhibitor, morphine had a significantly reduced effect on their flinch threshold. Both strains responded similarly with respect to the attenuation, induced by *p*-chlorophenylalanine, of the effects of challenging doses of morphine on rats made tolerant to the opiate by chronic administration in the form of implanted pellets, but once again it was the Sprague-Dawley rats that showed the greatest protection by the serotonin inhibitor against the effects of naloxone, the morphine antagonist mentioned above. The authors emphasized the importance of strain differences in the understanding of the role of *p*-chlorophenylalanine as a serotonin depletor and suggested that its use had revealed the Sprague-Dawley strain as one with an especially well-functioning brain serotonin system.

Gebhart and Mitchell (1973) were also concerned with the relationships of brain serotonin to the analgesic effects of morphine. They used the hot-plate apparatus in which the time taken to raise the feet, usually to lick them, was measured not in rats but mice. Two strains, unfamiliar in the present context, the CF1 and the CFW, were used, because the former is known to display a lower brain serotonin. While the hypothesis that the difference would lead to lower sensitivity to analgesic effects of morphine was not supported, and there were no differences between them in the development of tolerance to the drug, a drug-strain interaction in initial sensitivity was reported. At 2.0 mg/kg morphine sulfate, injected subcutaneously 30 min before testing, there was no difference between the strains, whereas a 4.0-mg/kg dose protected the CF1 mice significantly more, as determined by increased reaction times over control (saline) values. A determination of the doses required to allow 50% of those tested at a particular level to remain for 30 sec on the hot plate without reacting was also accomplished, and this confirmed the strain difference.

Reinhard *et al.* (1976) investigated other biogenic amines, dopamine and norepinephrine, as modified by morphine. Mice of four strains, C57BL/6J, BALB/6J, CD-1, and a Dublin Swiss strain were implanted subcutaneously with morphine pellets and the jump response to injections of naloxone was assessed 72 hr later. The C57 mice were shown to be markedly more sensitive than the BALB and Swiss mice, the CD-1 group being the least sensitive. Similarly, the C57 mice were the only ones to show a significant change in brain catecholamines in response to morphine; their norepinephrine levels in the striatal section assayed (comprising the corpora striata, hypothalamus, thalamus, and some midbrain and cortex) were significantly below control values. No other strains showed this effect and none showed changes in dopamine levels. When such determinations were made subsequently for three of the strains, that is, after naloxone treatment, the BALB now being omitted, only the Dublin Swiss mice showed a significant elevation of dopamine, as compared with saline controls. But none of these or other differences could be related to behavioral sensitivity.

Castellano *et al.* (1975) extended the approach by using mice of the familiar C57BL/6J and DBA/2J strains and pretesting them, before administering morphine, in ways designed to modify the known strain differences in brain biochemistry. Thus, in addition to the use of agents that interfered with adrenergic and cholinergic mediators, septal brain lesions were also used since they are known to decrease brain acetylcholine in related regions. Both kinds of environmental manipulation were shown to be effective by doses of 5, 10, and 20 mg/kg of morphine hydrochloride given intraperitoneally to lesioned and sham operated controls 30 min before exposure to the hot-plate test as described above. Drug–strain and lesion–strain interactions were demonstrated in that the DBA mice were more sensitive to the protective effects of morphine, which was reduced in both strains by the brain lesions. Recovery from the effects of morphine as observed by repeated testing at 60, 120, and 360 min showed a similar drug–strain interaction, with the DBA mice retaining the protective effect longer than the C57 group. Pretreatment, of intact mice only, with *a*-methyl-*p*-tyrosine, an inhibitor of noradrenaline synthesis, or with tranylcypromine, a monoamine oxidase inhibitor, 3 hr beforehand had no effect. Behavioral observations were widened to include motor activity as measured in the toggle cage apparatus described in Chapter 8, in order to study the so-called running fit induced by opiates, which may be independent in its action from the analgesia they typically induce. Here again a strain-limited effect of morphine was evident in that C57 mice increased activity in a dose-dependent fashion in a 30-min test, whereas the DBA were unaffected. Lesions had no significant effects. The effects of the pharmacological pretreatment, on the other hand, were evident in that while α-methyl-*p*-tyrosine uniformly blocked the increase of activity attributable to morphine, the effect of tranylcypromine was limited to the DBA mice, among which it abolished activity after morphine almost entirely—a finding the more remarkable since its effect when given alone was, at the two higher doses of the three used (1.25, 2.5, and 5.0 mg/kg), to increase activity in the toggle box in this strain. The findings relating to the C57 mice were confirmed by the results of Shuster *et al.* (1975*a*), who showed that this strain was far more responsive to 25 mg/kg of morphine sulfate than another, in this case, the A/J, in a similar test of locomotor activity by means of light-beam interruptions automatically monitored by photoelectric cells. An F_1 cross between the strains was intermediate, indicative of the absence of any marked degree of potence, an important point in connection with any effort to establish the genetic architecture of response to this drug.

Oliverio and Castellano (1974) extended the range of opiates studied from morphine only to include heroin, and from two strains to three, namely, C57BL/6J, DBA/2J, and BALB/cJ, though no crosses were made. Acute reaction to 5, 10, and 20 mg/kg of morphine injected intraperitoneally 30 min before testing varied with strain as seen in their dose-modulated increase in activity as measured in the toggle cage, but was lower if previous injections of the drug had been given, that is, tolerance was demonstrated. Hot-plate analgesia measured directly after injection also showed the same effect, but the ordering of the strains in the significant drug–strain interaction detected was different, BALB and DBA now being jointly the most sensitive to the drug and so giving longer latencies (slower responses), as opposed to the marked increase in measured activity shown by the C57, followed by the BALB with the DBA responding but little. These data are indicative of a dissociation in the two effects. Heroin, given in the same dose range as morphine (5, 10, and 20 mg/kg), gave similar values to morphine on the test of analgesia, no data on its effects on activity being presented. This omission was remedied (Castellano *et al.*, 1976) in an investigation which, while reverting to two strains, C57BL/6J and DBA/2J, increased the range of drugs studied to include amphetamine sulfate (2.0 mg/kg), strychnine nitrate (0.3 mg/kg), and ethanol (1.0 g/kg), given alone and in combination with heroin hydrochloride (5.0 mg/kg), intraperitoneally, in the doses indicated. Injections were given 15 min before toggle-cage activity was observed, except for heroin for which an interval of 30 min was used. While heroin combinations with amphetamine and with ethanol gave rise to significant increases in activity over heroin-alone values in the DBA strain, it was only the contribution with strychnine that gave a similar effect in the C57 strain. This marked drug–strain interaction is, however, complicated by the absence of significant effects of any of the significant elevations in toggle-cage activity to both amphetamine and heroin. Santos *et al.* (1973) briefly reported on the differential reactions of these same two strains, the C57BL/6J and DBA/2J, to sustained exposure to methadone. The former showed higher activity in the open field, but not the elevation of norepinephrine shown by the latter.

Collins *et al.* (1977) also report on the effects of morphine, again using the hot-plate apparatus. Seven strains of mice were studied, but the brief report concentrated largely on the effects of test experience and the development of tolerance after repeated administration. The presence of drug–strain interaction for the analgesia phenotype was reported, but not for a measure of activity.

Three of the four rat strains so far mentioned in this chapter, excluding the Fischer, were used by Borgen *et al.* (1970) in an observational study of aggressive behavior among groups of six rats after a 15-day regimen of increasing daily doses of morphine. The Sprague–Dawley group showed the least increase in fighting as compared with controls, the Wistars more, and the Long–Evans strain the most. The absence of statistical analysis renders these findings suggestive only, but the congruence with other work cited of the relative positions of the Sprague–Dawleys in the comparisons is of interest in that it would seem to support the view that features of their brain biochemistry render them less sensitive to the effects of morphine. Mention here may be made of a study also involving a form of aggressive behavior in the rat, mouse killing, which can be initiated by pilocarpine in rats that do not spontaneously show muricide. But, as Gay and Leaf (1976) have shown, the effect is strain dependent. They compared Holtzman albino rats with Long–Evans hooded ones and found that among both sexes there was a marked difference between them in response to 7.5 mg/kg injected intraperitoneally 15 min before exposure to a single mouse. While some 50% of the albino strain had killed after 12 such daily trials, very few of the hooded ones had, and dosages of 15.0 and 30.0 mg/kg were required to obtain comparable results. The cholinomimetic arecoline had no effect on either strain, which suggests a rather specific action for pilocarpine.

In one of the few studies of strain differences in preference behavior using morphine which has come to hand (Meade *et al.*, 1973), Wistar rats were compared with hooded ones of unspecified strain with respect to their response to the forced intake of morphine hydrochloride or morphine sulfate, both of which proved aversive to the former strain but not to the latter. Horowitz (1976) briefly reported that unlike other strains C57/6J mice will self-administer morphine in lethal doses when given with saccharin, and Whitney *et al.* (1977), in a similarly brief report, commented on the progress of work employing six inbred mouse strains. Positive preference between morphine masked with saccharin and water was shown to be highly correlated with increased activity in response to injection of morphine.

But none of these studies nor any of the ones employing morphine previously cited do more than lay the groundwork for biometrical analyses of the quantitative inheritance doubtless underlying responses to this drug. Only recently have any forms of genetical analysis been attempted, and of these, that by Eriksson and Kiianmaa (1971) takes pride of place. They used mice in a study closely tied to that of Eriksson (1971a) in that it employed the same C57BL and CBA inbred strains, in the same classical Mendelian breeding pattern in complete form, including backcrosses. Following a regimen that Nichols and Hsiao (1967) used for the rat (see Chapter 3), daily injections of morphine hydrochloride were given to the mice before they were offered a free choice between water and an aqueous solution of 0.5 mg/ml of morphine. As with their alcohol preference, the females of the C57BL mice showed a more marked preference than did the males, a difference not found in the generally lower-preference DBA mice or in any of the derived generations, except the F_1. The absence of reciprocal differences, that is, between the offspring of C57BL fathers and CBA mothers, and those with the parental strains reversed, which are indicative of maternal effects, enables such environmental effects to be discounted. But the biometrical analyses applied to the data are broadly unsatisfactory due to scalar problems not apparently amenable to the kind of data transformation applied with some success elsewhere in Eriksson's work (1971a) to avoid the complications of genotype–environment interaction—an outcome indicated by the scaling tests appropriately applied to the data. Little reliance can therefore be placed on the results of the analyses reported, which include values for heritability coefficients, beyond the observation that the phenotypic values would suggest a degree of dominance for high preference for morphine, though the cautions about the uncertainties involved in this kind of deduction from phenotype to genotype apply with full force in this as in every case.

The same observations might be made about the more limited approach to biometrical analysis of morphine-induced analgesia and activity offered by Castellano and Oliverio (1975) on the basis of a rather extensive breeding program. They used an incomplete 3×3 diallel cross design, employing the C57BL/6J, BALB/cJ, and DBA/2J strains but omitting the reciprocal crosses between the last two strains which the complete design requires. Backcrosses from the F_1 generation, which were bred to the appropriate parental strains, were, however, made, that is, again omitting combinations involving both BALB and DBA. Latency of response to thermal pain in the hot-plate test and activity in the toggle cage were determined under three doses of morphine hydrochloride, 5, 10, and 20 mg/kg, injected intraperitoneally before testing, in the same way as before (Oliverio and Castellano, 1974)—indeed, though not stated, the data for the parental strains were the same as those reported before, as may be seen from a comparison of Figures 1 and 2 in the earlier paper with Figures 1 and 3 in the later one. Not surprisingly, therefore, the findings relating to the parental

strains were identical, but interest centers on the filial and backcross generations. After the application of scaling tests (Mather and Jinks, 1971), which
showed that the phenotypic scales used were adequate for biometrical
analysis, it is disappointing to note that these were attempted in terms of
Bruell's (1962) genetic triangles. Once again it must be said that the power
inherent in the diallel crossbreeding design—albeit an incomplete one—is
unrealized by a piecemeal strain-by-strain approach to analyses based on
visual graphings and their associated formulas. Nevertheless, the data are of
considerable interest for the demonstration of the absence of reciprocal differences for either measure and for the demonstration of potence
(phenotypic dominance) for the higher, C57-like, activity response to morphine seen in crosses involving this strain. The backcross data for this
measure allow greater confidence that the phenotypic responses observed
may indeed reflect underlying directional dominance of the genes governing
this response, but only a more adequate analysis would allow certainty on
this point. As for the analgesia (hot–plate) latencies, the situation is less
clear since the backcross values were not presented and the most that can be
said is that F_1 hybrids show potence for the low sensitivity to the drug
demonstrated by the C57 mice.

We now turn to a series of studies concerned with the genetics of
behavioral response to morphine, which have used the techniques of recombinant inbred strains discussed earlier in Chapter 8. They are included in
summary Table XIII and are reviewed by Shuster (1975), who concludes
that ". . . a good start has been made (in defining) the genetic determinants
that control the response to narcotic drugs in mice" (p. 94), a conclusion
that depends largely for its acceptance on the reliance that can be placed on
the efficacy of the methodology used. To start at a fundamental level,
Baran *et al.* (1975) sought to determine the concentration in the brain of
mice of specific receptors that have been demonstrated to combine revers-
ibly with narcotics and their antagonists. This was done by ascertaining the
amount of binding of radioactive naloxone to opiate receptors in whole-
brain homogenates in the seven RI strains, together with the progenitor
strains and the F_1 crosses between them, a total of 11 in all. Two of the RI
strains formed outliers, high and low, and were significantly different from
an intermediate group that contained the rest of the strains, including the
progenitors. This being the case it was not possible to derive a strain
distribution pattern to pursue the analysis in the way previously described.
Baran *et al.* also measured analgesic behavior in response to an intraperitoneal injection of 5 mg/kg of morphine sulfate. Thermal pain was
again the stimulus but the response used was the tail flick, whose latency
was determined at 30, 60, 90, and 120 min after treatment. A rank-order
correlation for the strains between an integrated behavioral measure from
this test and the data on receptors was reported as $+0.48$, which, though
nonsignificant, comprehends the fact that one of the two outlier strains for

receptors was also extremely low in sensitivity to morphine. The same relationship did not hold, however, for the other, and no RI analysis was attempted for analgesia using these data. Shuster *et al.* (1975*b*) filled this gap, again using the tail-flick response, and adding a measure of running activity derived from photoelectric counter measurements. The same 11 strains of mice were tested, and the undrugged response to thermal pain was first investigated. As may be seen from the tabulation of the data provided by Shuster (1975, Table I), three groups, significantly differentiated from each other, may be formed from these basic latency data. Unfortunately, however, not one but two congener strains resembled the progenitor strain, the C57BL, in the intermediate grouping, which rendered the identification of the possible linkage of the tentative strain distribution pattern indeterminate. Response to three doses of morphine, 2.5, 5.0, and 10.0 mg/kg, measured at the same time intervals as before, produced a picture of some complexity with no clear-cut groupings, no relationship with initial, nondrugged values and, incidentally, no connection with pigmentation differences between the strains. Once again the methodology could not be pursued. For the activity phenotype, measured over 2 hr in response to 12.5, 25.0, and 40.0 mg/kg, averaging of the mean activity scores for all doses produced a tripartite grouping at the 60-min interval, which yielded a strain distribution pattern that could be accounted for in terms of a two-gene model. A different grouping of similar data at the 75-min interval was congruent with a single-gene model, but in neither case was there any linkage evidence from congener strains for either of the putative sets of loci. It is perhaps noteworthy that the possibility this implied of the differences in genetic architecture for essentially the same phenotypic measure at different time intervals after the initiation of its observation is one that can well be accepted since Wilcock and Fulker's demonstration (1973) of the existence of a change in the kind of genetic control of escape-avoidance conditioning with progressive trials.

Oliverio *et al.* (1975*b*) provided valuable replication of the above work using the same genetic methodology, but slightly different techniques of measurement, the toggle box for activity and the hot plate for analgesia. For activity, two doses (10 and 20 mg/kg) of morphine hydrochloride were given, 15 min before a 30-min observation period. The data show rather complex groupings, especially at the 10-mg/kg dose, which involved four major groupings. No strain distribution patterns were identified, though it was noted that probably more than two loci were involved. For analgesia 5, 10, and 20 mg/kg were given 30 min before the first test, others following at 30-min intervals up to 2 hr. No groupings were discussed but it was noted that the strain distribution pattern obtained was different from that of Shuster *et al.* (1975*b*), who, however, reported for this measure that ". . . it was difficult to discern a distinctive SDP for arriving at possible linkage" (p. 251). Nevertheless a significant interstudy correlation of $+0.77$ between strains when hot-plate and tail-flick analgesia are compared is impressive evidence for the stability of the phenotype, measured somewhat differently in different laboratories. Finally, Oliverio and his co-workers reported an ambitious attempt to unravel the genetics of tolerance to morphine, by comparing the scores on the hot-plate test of mice when made tolerant to morphine by five successive administrations over two days with their own original responses at the same doses as subsequently used. The data displayed a ". . . rather complex statistical overlap which hindered clarification and derivation of a genetic system" (p. 222), though it was later suggested that "The strain distribution pattern for tolerance indicated that a number of loci larger than possibly three was responsible. . ." (p. 223).

Thus the attempts to apply the recombinant inbred strain methodology to morphine phenotypes have encountered severe difficulties, and have thrown up definite indications of the polygenic nature of the genetic control of the phenotypes concerned, which, of course, the methodology is ill-equipped to handle. Only if the effect of major genes can be unequivocally identified can the techniques be crowned with the kind of success claimed in some of the investigations discussed earlier, and this achievement must, of course, be subject to replication and verification elsewhere before the existence of major genes governing drug responsivity of various kinds be accepted. But the work reviewed has been of considerable interest and utility. The absence of reciprocal cross differences, for example, which the data generally reveal, is reassuring since it points away from prenatal maternal effects or sex linkage as being potential problems in this area, and there have been examples of rather clear demonstrations of potence and its absence, which will be of interest for future workers.

Finally, these C57BL and DBA strains also figure in reports by Belknap *et al.* (1973) of the induction of dependence on phenobarbital by feeding them the drug in the diet for six days. In contrast with mice of the DBA strain, the C57 mice consumed more phenobarbital per unit of body weight, though it is not possible from the data presented to know if this finding represents a preference—either pharmacological or taste—or not. But what is clear is that observational tests of intoxication including motor incoordination show that they are also more resistant to the drug, as well as being less prone to seizure and other symptoms during the period after the abrupt withdrawal of the drug from the diet. As in Goldstein's (1973) work the seizure phenomena were observed after withdrawal, reaching a peak somewhat later, however, at 22–36 hr and declining thereafter. These findings have been confirmed by Belknap *et al.* (1976) and extended by Cocke and Belknap (1976), who showed that both strains' withdrawal symptoms could be exacerbated by a magnesium-deficient diet. Once again the basis for pharmacogenetic analysis has been laid, but no more. These experiments are summarized in Table XVII, together with those cited on work with opiates—except for experimentation using the recombinant inbred strain methodology, which, as already noted, are included in Table XIII.

TABLE XVII

Psychopharmacogenetic Experiments with Opiates and Barbiturates

Reference	Species (and strain)	Treatment	Measure	Outcome	Remarks
Way *et al.* (1969), Brase *et al.* (1974)	Mouse, morphine addicted	Naloxone injection	Hyperalgesic jumping	Strain differences	
Sinclair *et al.* (1973)	Rat, Wistar albino, Long–Evans hooded	Morphine	Ethanol preference suppression	No strain difference	
Tilson and Rech (1974)	Rat, Fischer, Sprague–Dawley	Morphine and naloxone	Flinch threshold to shock	Drug–strain interaction Sprague–Dawley threshold elevated by morphine and Sprague–Dawleys most protected by *p*-chlor-phenylalanine	
Gebhart and Mitchell (1973)	Mouse, CF1, CFW	Morphine sulfate	Latency to raise foot on hot plate	Drug–strain interaction for initial sensitivity to drug. CF1 protected more. No strain difference in tolerance	
Castellano *et al.* (1975)	Mouse, C57BL/6J, DBA/2J	Morphine hydrochloride	Hot plate	Drug–strain and lesion–strain interactions found. DBA more sensitive to protection by drug. Drug–strain interaction in recovery effects also	

(Continued)

TABLE XVII—*Continued*

Reference	Species (and strain)	Treatment	Measure	Outcome	Remarks
Castellano *et al.* (1975) *(continued)*			Activity in toggle cage	C57 but not DBA showed dose-dependent increase	
		Morphine hydrochloride with *a*-methyl-*p*-tyrosine Tranylcypromine		Blocked morphine-induced activity Blocked DBA activity but not C57	
Shuster *et al.* (1975*a*)	Mouse, C57, A/J and F₁ cross	Morphine sulfate	Activity, automatically recorded	C57 more responsive than DBA to drug	
Reinhard *et al.* (1976)	Mouse, C57BL/6J, BALB/6J, CD-1, Dublin Swiss	Morphine	Dopamine level Norepinephrine level Jump response to naloxone	No significant change C57 significant change C57 most sensitive, CD-1 least	
Oliverio and Castellano (1974)	Mouse, C57BL/6J, DBA/2J, BALB/cJ	Morphine	Activity in toggle cage. Hot-plate analgesia	Strain differences and tolerance shown. Drug–strain interaction but patterning different	Dissociation of effects indicated
Santos *et al.* (1973)	Mouse, C57BL/6J, DBA/2J	Heroin Methadone	Hot-plate analgesia Open-field activity	As morphine C57BL > DBA DBA showed raised norepinephrine	
Collins *et al.* (1977)	Mouse, 7 strains	Morphine	Hot-plate analgesia Activity	Drug–strain interaction No drug–strain interaction	
Borgen *et al.* (1970)	Rat, Sprague-Dawley, Wistar, Long-Evans hooded, and controls	Morphine	Aggression (observational)	Long-Evans > Wistar > control > Sprague-Dawley	No statistical analysis

Reference	Species, strain	Drug	Measure	Results	Comments
Gay and Leaf (1976)	Rat, Holtzman albino, Long-Evans hooded	Pilocarpine Arecoline	Muricide Muricide	Increases for albinos only No effect on either strain No effect on either strain.	
Meade et al. (1973)	Rat, Wistar, hooded	Morphine hydrochloride or morphine sulfate	Preference	Drugs aversive to Wistars only	
Horowitz (1976)	Mouse, C57/6J, and others	Morphine with saccharin	Self-administration intake	Only C57/6J take lethal doses	Brief report
Whitney et al. (1977)	Mouse, 6 strains	Morphine with saccharin	Preference	Preference correlated with morphine-induced activity	Brief report
Eriksson and Kiianmaa (1971)	Mouse, C57BL, DBA, and crosses and backcrosses	Morphine hydrochloride daily pretreatment	Preference	Female C57BL > male, dominance for morphine preference	Similar results for alcohol Unsatisfactory analyses
Castellano and Oliverio (1975)	Mouse, C57BL/6J, BALB/cJ, DBA/2J, and crosses and backcrosses	Morphine hydrochloride daily pretreatment	Activity	Potence and (?) directional dominance for high-morphine-induced activity	Incomplete diallel. Unsatisfactory analyses
			Hot-plate analgesia	F_1 showed potence for low sensitivity of C57	Data less fully reported
Belknap et al. (1973)	Mouse, C57BL, DBA	Phenobarbital	Phenobarbital ingestion (after prefeeding) Motor incoordination Seizure after withdrawal	C57 consumed more C57 more resistant Confirmed Goldstein (1973)	Further confirmed by Belknap et al. (1976) and Cocke and Belknap (1976)
Castellano et al. (1976)	Mouse, C57BL/6J, DBA/2J	Amphetamine, strychnine, ethanol alone and with heroin	Toggle-cage activity	Drug-strain interaction	

As adumbrated earlier, the study of alcohol preference, response to opiates, and similar phenotypes has generated work of considerable interest, leading to some of the most advanced biometrical analyses based on strain differences in both mice and rats, the latter based especially on selected strains. But, once again, it must be concluded that generalizations regarding the genetic architecture of the phenotypes are far from clear and the evolutionary implications that can flow from it consequently far from secure. The discrepancy between the various analyses of directional dominance for preference in the mouse referred to above exemplify the rudimentary nature of the foundations upon which the inferences from genetic structure to adaptive significance are built in psychopharmacogenetics.

While these discrepancies are cause for comment, they need not be cause for undue concern. The acceptance of the need for adequate analyses of behavioral phenotypes into their environmental and genetic components and their respective subdivisions is far from complete in this area of psychology as in any other and psychopharmacology presents its own special complexities, as we have seen. Only when adequately designed and—perhaps more important—appropriately analyzed animal experimentation is the norm rather than the exception can we expect to make significant progress. As we have constantly observed during the course of this review, the groundwork has been laid time and again: Plans, sometimes competing, for the superstructure are being advanced, as in this review, but the edifice has yet to be built.

Chapter 10

Overview

Throughout this book an emphasis has been laid on the biometrical genetical approach to the problems of unravelling the various determinants of individual differences in drug response. This bias, if such it be, will have been evident to the reader who was, indeed, warned of it at the outset (see Chapter 1). No apology therefore seems to be called for for this emphasis. On the contrary, it has provided the writer with a vantage point from which to view the contemporary literature with a consistency of approach hitherto not a conspicuous feature of the analysis of the dependence of drug effects on genetic background. But the applications of the principles underlying this approach have been dealt with piecemeal as they have arisen so that the importance of those principles themselves may have been obscured by the details of the contexts in which they have appeared. It seems desirable, therefore, to review them, in a series of summary and hence somewhat didactic statements (Broadhurst and Jinks, 1977) before proceeding briefly to assess, in each case, the extent to which the material reviewed in this book illustrates them. It will be seen that most of the programmatic points to be developed have been referred to earlier, though not necessarily in the order given. Sometimes, indeed, they go beyond the review, usually because relevant examples have not been encountered in the psychopharmacological literature. In other cases the examples which could be adduced do not especially illuminate the extent to which the biometrical approach can be utilized in their analysis. Often experiments were not planned in such a way as to render them potentially amenable to appropriate analysis of this kind. In other cases, while the data appear satisfactory, the analysis brought to bear on them is less powerful than biometrical methods allow.

The first point to note is that individual differences in drug responsivity are multidetermined both environmentally and genetically. An adequate analysis of their effects as seen in the behavior of animals and attributable to the effects of drugs includes, therefore, consideration of both heritable and nonheritable sources of variation. The techniques of biometrical genetics, though largely derived from plant investigations, can be applied to behavioral phenotypes with advantage, and in this respect the psychopharmacological field is no different from any other. This is the central tenet of all forms of quantitative genetic analysis and the numerous examples of drug–strain interaction noted in this book are a potent reminder of the essential nature of this proposition. Second, the biometrical approach recognizes causation as heritable (genetic) and nonheritable (environmental), the latter including internal effects such as those of drugs. The interaction both between and within these two major classes is recognized as contributing to the observed, phenotypic variation as well. This principle carries matters somewhat further in that it asserts that the biometrical models employed in the analysis of phenotypic variation are explicitly concerned with apportioning the observed variation between the two major components putatively determining that variation. Those major components are themselves subject to further subdivision, additive, dominance, and epistatic variation being the principle classes of heritable variation commonly identified and, on the environmental side, the possibilities are numerous. Perhaps maternal effects are the environmental effect most typically encountered in such analyses. In principle, however, the whole range of causative agents recognized by behavioral workers and relating to stimulus changes ranging from subtle husbandry variables on the one hand to explicit treatment variables on the other are amenable to such analysis. Examples of the former are to be found in the work of Vesell *et al.* (1976) cited in Chapter 1, and of the latter in numerous cases in which the response to a drug has been manipulated by prior treatment, such as the intensity of withdrawal symptoms elicited by naloxone after pretreatment with morphine, discussed in Section 9.2. In this way the constituents of the phenotype can be teased apart, and the importance of the various contributions to the multidetermined effects assessed. The interactive effects of these constituents is of considerable interest and the numerous drug–strain interactions mentioned above and observed at the phenotypic level give good ground for suspecting that genotype–environment interactions may be important interactive determinants when the data are considered at a more analytic level. No unequivocal examples can be cited from the work reviewed, but the need for biometrical models that allow the estimation of such effects will become apparent when appropriate analyses come to be undertaken. Even more remote, perhaps, is the possibility of analyzing phenotypic drug responses in terms of the interactive components recognized as contibuting to within-genotypic effects, as opposed to the between genetic and environmental determinants of the kind just discussed. In addition to dominance variation, which itself may be unidirectional or ambidirectional and which is essentially an allelic effect, there is a class of nonallelic interactions, subsumed under the term epistasis. Biometrical genetics recognizes three principal classes, i-type, j-type, and l-type, relating respectively to interaction between uniformly homozygous, uniformly heterozygous, and mixed homozygous–heterozygous gene combinations. It may well be some time before such effects are identified as contributing to psychopharmacological phenotypic variation.

In connection with the model fitting implied in the preceding paragraph, it should also be noticed that the biometrical approach involves a concern with the adequacy of the scale of measurement, so that the interactions between the different kinds of genetical variation on the one hand (nonallelic interaction) and between genetical and environmental variation (genotype–environment interaction) can be detected and, if shown to be necessary, minimized. In this way biometrical models of a greater simplicity may be fitted, without the need for more data from, for example, different filial or backcross generations, which an inadequate scale might necessitate. Transformation of raw data may therefore be appropriate as a first stage to the analysis of first- and second-degree statistics. No examples have been encountered in the psychopharmacogenetical literature reviewed in this monograph. Other impediments to efficient analysis are environmental maternal effects and sex linkage of genes, both of which are perturbations to be reckoned with but which can be accommodated within a biometrical model and their effects assessed. As yet only Eriksson (1969a) has been innovative enough to invoke sex linkage as an explanatory mechanism, but, as we have seen (Chapter 3), the evidence is not strong.

Techniques of proven applicability in the psychogenetic analysis of behavioral phenotypes include selection, parent–offspring correlational analysis, the classical crossing of inbred strains and the rearing of first- and of second-filial and backcross generations, the diallel cross—the method of complete intercrossing of several strains—and triple-test crossing methods. A wealth of examples of the utility of selection as a technique applied to behavioral pharmacology has been described, and examples of the use of parent–offspring correlation included those of Whitney *et al.* (1970; Section 9.2) and of Murphree (1973; see Chapter 4), but most of the analyses of data gathered in these ways have been disappointing. Mendelian crosses have also been ubiquitous, and the attempts at the analysis of their outcome more sophisticated, especially in the hands of McClearn and his group, but as yet their use in the analysis of drug responsivity as a phenotype lags behind that of other behavioral responses. Similarly, the diallel cross design has not been used to maximal efficiency, and the triple-test cross, as yet, not at all. On the other hand, the use of recombinant inbred strains to detect the effect of major genes has been largely limited to psychopharmacology, but the technique has considerable difficulties and is yet to prove of decisive advantage. While the number of genes or groups of genes involved in determining a given phenotype can be estimated, the only example of this approach in psychopharmacology is the somewhat less than positive one arrived at by Oliverio *et al.* (1973*a*), who concluded (see Chapter 8) that the variation due to amphetamine was insusceptible of analysis by their methods of recombinant inbred strains and strain distribution pattern analysis and hence is polygenic in character. The implication that it is therefore also unanalyzable is one which the whole of the present approach seeks to challenge.

It is now widely understood that the term heritability refers to a convenient index expressing the ratio of the genetic to the total variation of a behavioral response in a given population, and several examples of its use are cited in this monograph. What is perhaps less widely recognized is that it is the end point of an adequate genetical analysis, not its beginning. For example, only when the additive and dominance components contributing to the genetical variation have been reliably distinguished can the two types of heritability ratio ("broad" and "narrow") be discriminated, since in the former the dominance component is aggregated in the numerator whereas in the latter it is excluded. When such distinctions are made, through the efficient analysis of phenotypic variation, this and other subtleties of the genetic architecture mentioned above—directionality of dominance, presence and kind of epistasis—will afford the possibility of speculative attempts to understand how behavioral responses to drugs have evolved, in the way that has been done for other behavior phenotypes (Broadhurst and Jinks, 1974). Michelson's account (1974) provides an example of what can be achieved, albeit by other than biometrical methods, in understanding at the biochemical level the development of the chemical sensitivity of tissues and organs during evolution.

Finally, heterosis ("hybrid vigor") should be mentioned. It is a complex phenomenon primarily due to genetic interactions whose effect can be assessed, and expresses itself in phenotypic values in first filial crosses, which transcend those of the parents; that is to say, phenotypic dominance (termed "potence" for reasons already rehearsed—see Chapter 6) is particularly marked, meriting the attribution of "overdominance." Examples were cited in connection with the reports by Anisman on his analyses using the diallel cross method (Chapter 6), but, as noted in the discussion of that work, the analyses employed lacked power to demonstrate unequivocally the genetic mechanisms involved. But the biometrical model can be further elaborated to analyze situations of a far greater degree of complexity than has yet been required in psychopharmacology. This is merely one example in an area in which experimentation has lagged behind theory to a degree bordering on the spectacular.

This conclusion underlines what has been said earlier: Since the awareness of the importance of heritable variation in psychopharmacology is itself of relatively recent standing, it is not remarkable that the assimilation of techniques to evaluate its quantitative aspects necessarily trails conspicuously. But the message is now clear—such techniques do exist and they can be applied. If this whole survey has done no more than alert the reader to these possibilities, then it will have served a useful purpose.

References

Abel, E. L., 1975, Emotionality in offspring of rats fed alcohol while nursing, *J. Stud. Alcohol* **36**:654-658.

Ahtee, L., 1972, The metabolism of brain 5-hydroxytryptamine in rat strains selected for alcohol preference or rejection: Effects of ethanol, in *International Symposium Biological Aspects of Alcohol Consumption 27-29 September 1971,* Vol. 20 (O. Forsander and K. Eriksson, eds.), pp. 193-199, Finnish Foundation for Alcohol Studies, Helsinki.

Ahtee, L., and Eriksson, E., 1972, 5-hydroxytryptamine and 5-hydroxyindolylacetic acid content in brain of rat strains selected for their alcohol intake, *Physiol. Behav.* **8**:123-126.

Ahtee, L., and Eriksson, K., 1973, Regional distribution of brain 5-hydroxytryptamine in rat strains selected for their alcohol intake, *Ann. N. Y. Acad. Sci.* **215**:126-134.

Ahtee, L., and Eriksson, K., 1975, Dopamine and noradrenaline content in the brain of rat strains selected for their alcohol intake, *Acta Physiol. Scand.* **93**:563-565.

Amit, Z., Levitan, D. E., and Lindros, K. O., 1976, Suppression of ethanol intake following administration of dopamine-beta-hydroxylase inhibitors in rats, *Arch. Int. Pharmac. Therap.* **223**:114-119.

Anderson, S. M., and McClearn, G. E., 1975, Ethanol acceptance under thirst motivation and hepatic enzymes in mice, *Behav. Genet.* **5**:87-88 (abstract).

Angel, C., Murphree, O. D., and DeLuca, D. C., 1974, The effects of chlordiazepoxide, amphetamine and cocaine on bar-press behavior in normal and genetically nervous dogs, *Dis. Nerv. Syst.* **35**:220-223.

Anisman, H., 1975a, Differential effects of scopolamine and D-amphetamine on avoidance: Strain interactions, *Pharmacol. Biochem. Behav.* **3**:809-817.

Anisman, H., 1975b, Dissociation of disinhibitory effects of scopolamine: Strain and task factors, *Pharmacol. Biochem. Behav.* **3**:613-618.

Anisman, H., 1975c, Effects of scopolamine and *d*-amphetamine on one-way shuttle, and inhibitory avoidance: A diallel analysis in mice, *Pharmacol. Biochem. Behav.* **3**:1037-1042.

Anisman, H., 1975d, Time-dependent variations in aversively motivated behaviors: Non-associative effects of cholinergic and catecholaminergic activity, *Psychol. Rev.* **82**:359-385.

Anisman, H., 1976a, Effects of scopolamine and *d*-amphetamine on locomotor activity before and after shock: A diallel analysis in mice, *Psychopharmacology* **48**:165-173.

Anisman, H., 1976b, Role of stimulus locale on strain differences in active avoidance after scopolamine or *d*-amphetamine treatment, *Pharmacol. Biochem. Behav.* **4**:103-106.

Anisman, H., and Cygan, D., 1975, Central effects of scopolamine and (+)-amphetamine on locomotor activity: Interaction with strain and stress variables, *Neuropharmacology* **14**:835-840.

Anisman, H., and Kokkinidis, L., 1975, Effects of scopolamine, *d*-amphetamine and other drugs affecting catecholamines on spontaneous alternation and locomotor activity in mice, *Psychopharmacologia* **45**:55-63.

Anisman, H., and Waller, T. G., 1974, Effects of inescapable shock and shock-produced conflict on self selection of alcohol in rats, *Pharmacol. Biochem. Behav.* **2**:27-34.

Anisman, H., Wahlsten, D., and Kokkinidis, L., 1975, Effects of *d*-amphetamine and scopolamine on activity before and after shock in three mouse strains, *Pharmacol. Biochem. Behav.* **3**:819-824.

Appel, S. H., 1965, Effect of inhibition of RNA synthesis on neural information storage, *Nature (London)* **207**:1163-1166.

Archer, J., 1975, The Maudsley reactive and nonreactive strains of rats: The need for an objective evaluation, *Behav. Genet.* **5**:411-413.

Baer, D. S., and Crumpacker, D. W., 1975, Effects of maternal ingestion of alcohol on maternal care and behavior of progeny in mice, *Behav. Genet.* **5**:88 (abstract).

Bailey, D. W., 1971, Recombinant-inbred strains: An aid to finding identity, linkage, and function of histocompatibility and other genes, *Transplantation* **11**:325-327.

Bailey, D. W., and Hoste, J., 1971, A gene governing the female immune response to the male antigen in mice, *Transplantation* **11**:404-407.

Baran, A., Shuster, L., Eleftheriou, B. E., and Bailey, D. W., 1975, Opiate receptors in mice: Genetic differences, *Life Sci.* **17**:633-640.

Barrett, R. J., Leith, N. J., and Ray, O. S., 1973, A behavioral and pharmacological analysis of variables mediating active-avoidance behavior in rats, *J. Comp. Physiol. Psychol.* **82**:489-500.

Bättig, K., Driscoll, P., Schlatter, J., and Uster, H. J., 1976, Effects of nicotine on the exploratory locomotion patterns of female Roman high- and low-avoidance rats, *Pharmacol. Biochem. Behav.* **4**:435-439.

Baum, M., 1971, Effect of alcohol on the resistance-to-extinction of an avoidance response: Replication in mice, *Physiol. Behav.* **6**:307-310.

Beckwith, B. E., Sandman, C. A., Alexander, W. D., Gerald, M. C., and Goldman, H., 1974, *d*-Amphetamine effects on attention and memory in the albino and hooded rat, *Pharmacol. Physiol. Behav.* **2**:557-561.

Belknap, J. K., 1977, The regulation of ethanol consumption (alcohol preference) in C57BL/6J and DBA/2J mice: Evidence for an orosensory component in the avoidance of ethanol by DBA/2J mice, *Behav. Genet.* **7**:43-44 (abstract).

Belknap, J. K., MacInnes, J. W., and McClearn, G. E., 1972, Ethanol sleep times and hepatic alcohol and aldehyde dehydrogenase activities in mice, *Physiol. Behav.* **9**:453-457.

Belknap, J. K., Waddingham, S., and Ondrusek, G., 1973, Barbiturate dependence in mice induced by a single short-term oral procedure, *Physiol. Psychol.* **1**:394-396.

Belknap, J. K., Ondrusek, G., and Waddingham, S., 1976, Barbiturate-induced physical dependence and functional tolerance development in inbred mice, *Behav. Genet.* **6**:9-10 (abstract).

Bignami, G., 1965, Selection for high rates and low rates of conditioning in the rat, *Anim. Behav.* **13**:221-227.

Bignami, G., and Bovet, D., 1965, Expérience de sélection par rapport à une réaction conditionnée d'évitement chez le rat, *C. R. Acad. Sci.* **260**:1239-1244.

Bignami, G., Robustelli, F., Janků, I., and Bovet, D., 1965, Action de l'amphétamine et de quelques agents psychotropes sur l'acquisition d'un conditionnement de fuite et d'évitement chez des rats selectionnés d'un niveau particulierèment bas de leurs performances, *C. R. Acad. Sci.* **260**:4273-4278.

Bliss, D. K., 1974, Theoretical explanations of drug-dissociated behaviors, *Fed. Proc., Fed. Am. Soc. Exp. Biol.* **33**:1787-1796.

Boggan, W. O., and Seiden L. S., 1971, Dopa reversal of reserpine enhancement of audiogenic seizure susceptibility in mice, *Physiol. Behav.* **6**:215-217.

Boggan, W. O., Freedman, D. X., Lovell, R. A., and Schlesinger, K., 1971, Studies in audiogenic seizure susceptibility, *Psychopharmacologia* **20**:48-56.

Boissier, J. R., Simon, P., and Soubrié, P., 1976, *New Approaches to the Study of Anxiety and Anxiolytic Drugs in Animals, Proceedings of the 6th International Congress of Pharmacology, Helsinki, 1975* (J. Tuomisto and M. K. Paasonen, eds.), pp. 213-222, Pergamon, Oxford.

Borgen, L. A., Khalsa, J. H., King, W. T., and Davis, W. M., 1970, Strain differences in morphine-withdrawal induced aggression in rats, *Psychon. Sci.* **21**:35-36.

Bourgault, P. C., Karczmar, A. G., and Scudder, C. L., 1963, Contrasting behavioral, pharmacological, neurophysiological, and biochemical profiles of C57 Bl/6 and SC-1 strains of mice, *Life Sci.* **8**:533-553.

Bovet, D., and Oliverio, A., 1967, Decrement of avoidance conditioning performance in inbred mice subjected to prolonged sessions: Performance recovery after rest and amphetamine, *J. Psychol.* **65**:45-55.

Bovet, D., and Oliverio, A., 1973, Pharmacogenetic aspects of learning and memory, in *Brain, Nerves and Synapses,* Vol. 4, *Pharmacology and the Future of Man, Proceedings of the Vth International Congress on Pharmacology, San Francisco, California, July 1972* (F. E. Bloom and G. H. Acheson, eds.), pp. 18-28, Karger, Basel.

Bovet, D., Bovet-Nitti, F., and Oliverio, A., 1966, Effects of nicotine on avoidance conditioning of inbred strains of mice, *Psychopharmacologia* **10**:1-5.

Bovet, D., Bovet-Nitti, F., and Oliverio, A., 1969, Genetic aspects of learning and memory in mice, *Science* **163**:139-149.

Bovet-Nitti, F., 1966, Facilitation of simultaneous visual discrimination by nicotine in the rat, *Psychopharmacologia* **10**:59-66.

Bovet-Nitti, F., 1969, Facilitation of simultaneous visual discrimination by nicotine in four "inbred" strains of mice, *Psychopharmacologia* **14**:193-199.

Bradley, D. W. M., Joyce, D., Murphy, E. H., Nash, B. M., Porsolt, R. D., Summerfield, A., and Twyman, W. A., 1968, Amphetamine–barbiturate mixture: Effects on the behaviour of mice, *Nature (London)* **220**:187-188.

Brase, D. A., Tseng, L. F., Loh, H. H., and Way, E. L., 1974, Cholinergic modification of naloxone-induced jumping in morphine dependent mice, *Eur. J. Pharmacol.* **26**:1-8.

Breen, R. A., and McGaugh, J. L., 1961, Facilitation of maze learning with posttrial injections of picrotoxin, *J. Comp. Physiol. Psychol.* **54**:498-501.

Brewster, D. J., 1968, Genetic analysis of ethanol preference in rats selected for emotional reactivity, *J. Hered.* **5**:283-285.

Brewster, D. J., 1969, Ethanol preference in strains of rats selectively bred for behavioral characteristics, *J. Genet. Psychol.* **115**:217-227.

Brewster, D. J., 1972, Ethanol preference in strains of rats selectively bred for behavioral characteristics, *Ann. N. Y. Acad. Sci.* **197**:49-53.

Brimblecombe, R. W., Buxton, D. A., and Redfern, P. H., 1975, Drug effects on avoidance behaviour in selected strains of rats, *Br. J. Pharmacol.* **53**:461P.

Broadhurst, P. L., 1958, Studies in psychogenetics: The quantitative inheritance of behaviour in rats investigated by selective and cross-breeding, *Bull. Br. Psychol. Soc.* **34**, 2A (abstract).

Broadhurst, P. L., 1960, Experiments in psychogenetics: Applications of biometrical genetics to the inheritance of behaviour, in: *Experiments in Personality,* Vol. I, *Psychogenetics and Psychopharmacology* (H.J. Eysenck, ed.), pp. 1-102, Routledge and Kegan Paul, London.

Broadhurst, P. L., 1961, Analysis of maternal effects in the inheritance of behaviour, *Anim. Behav.* 9:129-141.

Broadhurst, P. L., 1962, A note on further progress in a psychogenetic selection experiment, *Psychol. Rep.* 10:65-66.

Broadhurst, P. L., 1964, The hereditary base for the action of drugs on animal behaviour, in: *Animal Behaviour and Drug Action. Ciba Foundation Symposium Jointly with Co-ordinating Committee for Symposia on Drug Action* (H. Steinberg, A. V. S. de Reuck, and J. Knight, eds.), pp. 224-236, Churchill, London.

Broadhurst, P. L., 1968, Experimental approaches to the evolution of behavior, in: *Genetics and Environmental Influences on Behaviour. Eugenics Society Symposia,* Vol. 4 (J. M. Thoday and A. S. Parkes, eds.) pp. 15-36, Oliver and Boyd, Edinburgh.

Broadhurst, P. L., 1975, The Maudsley reactive and nonreactive strains of rats: A survey, *Behav. Genet.* 5:299-319.

Broadhurst, P. L., 1976, The Maudsley reactive and nonreactive strains of rats: A clarification, *Behav. Genet.* 6:363-365.

Broadhurst, P. L., 1977, Pharmacogenetics, in: *Handbook of Psychopharmacology,* Vol. 7, *Principles of Behavioral Pharmacology* (L. L. Iversen, S. D. Iversen, and S. H. Snyder, eds.), pp. 265-320, Plenum Press, New York.

Broadhurst, P. L., and Bignami, G., 1965, Correlative effects of psychogenetic selection: A study of the Roman high and low avoidance strains of rats, *Behav. Res. Ther.* 2:273-280.

Broadhurst, P. L., and Eysenck, H. J., 1965, Emotionality in the rat: A problem of response specificity, in: *Stephanos: Studies in Psychology Presented to Cyril Burt* (C. Banks and P. L. Broadhurst, eds.), pp. 205-222, University of London Press, London.

Broadhurst, P. L., and Jinks, J. L., 1974, What genetical architecture can tell us about the natural selection of behavioural traits, in: *The Genetics of Behaviour* (J. H. F. van Abeelen, ed.), pp. 43-63, North Holland Publishing Co., Amsterdam.

Broadhurst, P. L., and Jinks, J. L., 1977, Psychological genetics, from the study of animal behavior, in: *Handbook of Modern Personality Theory* (R. B. Cattell and R. M. Dreger, eds.), pp. 295-328, Hemisphere-Wiley, New York.

Broadhurst, P. L., and Wallgren, H., 1964, Ethanol and the acquisition of a conditioned avoidance response in selected strains of rats, *J. Stud. Alcohol* 25:476-489.

Broadhurst, P. L., Sinha, S. N., and Singh, S. D., 1959, The effect of stimulant and depressant drugs on a measure of emotional reactivity in the rat, *J. Genet. Psychol.* 95:217-226.

Broadhurst, P. L., Fulker, D. W., and Wilcock, J., 1974, Behavioral genetics, *Ann. Rev. Psychol.* 25:389-415.

Brodie, B. B., 1962, Drug metabolism—subcellular mechanisms, in: *Enzymes and Drug Action* (J. L. Mongar and A. V. S. de Reuck, eds.), pp. 317-343, Churchill, London.

Bruell, J. H., 1962, Dominance and segregation in the inheritance of quantitative behavior in mice, in: *Roots of Behavior* (E. Bliss, ed.), pp. 48-67, Harper Bros., New York.

Bruell, J. H., 1969, Genetics and adaptive significance of emotional defecation in mice, *Ann. N. Y. Acad. Sci.* 159:825-830.

Buckholtz, N. S., 1974, Shuttle-avoidance learning of mice: Effects of post-trial pentylenetetrazol, strain, and age, *Psychol. Rep.* 35:319-326.

Burt, G. S., 1962, Strain differences in picrotoxin seizure threshold, *Nature (London)* 193:301-302.

Busnel, R. G., and Lehmann, A., 1961, Action de convulsants chimiques sur des souris de lignées sensible et résistante à la crise audiogène, *J. Physiol. (Paris)* **53**:285-286.

Buxton, D. A., 1974, Cholinergic mechanism and behaviour in selected strains of rats, unpublished doctoral dissertation, University of Bath, England.

Buxton, D. A., Brimblecombe, R. W., French, M. C., and Redfern, P. H., 1976, Brain acetylcholine concentration and acetylcholinesterase activity in selectively-bred strains of rats, *Psychopharmacology* **47**:97-99.

Calhoun, W. H., 1965, The effect of strychnine sulphate on the home cage activity and oxygen consumption in three inbred strains of mice, *Psychopharmacologia* **8**:227-234.

Castellano, C., 1976, Effects of nicotine on discrimination learning, consolidation and learned behaviour in two inbred strains of mice, *Psychopharmacology* **48**:37-43.

Castellano, C., and Oliverio, A., 1975, A genetic analysis of morphine-induced running and analgesia in the mouse, *Psychopharmacologia* **41**:197-200.

Castellano, C., Eleftheriou, B. E., Bailey, D. W., and Oliverio, A., 1974, Chlorpromazine and avoidance: A genetic analysis, *Psychopharmacologia* **34**:309-316.

Castellano, C., Llovera, B. E., and Oliverio, A., 1975, Morphine-induced running and analgesia in two strains of mice following septal lesions or modification of brain amines, *Naunyn-Schmiedeberg's Arch. Pharmacol.* **288**:355-370.

Castellano, C., Filibeck, U., and Oliverio, A., 1976, Effects of heroin, alone or in combination with other drugs, on the locomotor activity in two inbred strains of mice, *Psychopharmacology* **49**:29-31.

Cazala, P., 1976, Effects of *d*- and *l*-amphetamine on dorsal and ventral hypothalamic self-stimulation in three inbred strains of mice, *Pharmacol. Biochem. Behav.* **5**:505-510.

Chan, A. W. K., 1976, Gamma aminobutyric acid in different strains of mice. Effect of ethanol, *Life Sci.* **19**:597-604.

Chance, M. R. A., 1946, Aggregation as a factor influencing the toxicity of sympathomimetic amines in mice, *J. Pharm. Exp. Ther.* **87**:214-219.

Church, A. C., 1977, Motor responses to a cute alcohol administration in mice selected for differential alcohol-induced sleep time, *Behav. Genet.* **7**:49 (abstract).

Church, A. C., 1977, Motor responses to acute alcohol administration in mice selected for selected for sensitivity to alcohol, *Psychopharmacology* **47**:49-52.

Cocke, R., and Belknap. J. K., 1976, Possible role of magnesium deficiency in the etiology of the barbiturate withdrawal syndrome in mice, *Behav. Genet.* **6**:103 (abstract).

Collins, A. C., and Deitrich, R. A., 1973, Alterations in catecholamine turnover by ethanol in lines of mice which differ in ethanol sleep time, *Behav. Genet.* **3**:398 (abstract).

Collins, R. L., 1964, Inheritance of avoidance conditioning in mice, *Science* **143**:1188-1190.

Collins, R. L., Horowitz, G. P., and Passe, D. H., 1977, Genotype and test experience as determinants of sensitivity and tolerance to morphine, *Behav. Genet.* **7**:50 (abstract).

Coyle, J. T., Jr., Wender, P., and Lipsky, A., 1973, Avoidance conditioning in different strains of rats: Neurochemical correlates, *Psychopharmacologia* **31**:25-34.

Damjanovich, R. P., and MacInnes, J. W., 1973, Factors involved in ethanol narcosis: Analysis in mice of three inbred strains, *Life Sci.* **13**:55-65.

Dantzer, R., 1974, De la psychopharmacologie à la psychopharmacogénétique. Déterminants des effets des drogues sur le comportement, rôle des facteurs génétiques, *Anné Psychol.* **74**:507-532.

Davis, W. M.. and King, W. T., 1967, Pharmacogenetic factor in the convulsive responses of mice to flurothyl, *Experientia* **23**:214-215.

Davis, W. M., and Webb, O. L., 1963, A circadian rhythm of chemoconvulsive response thresholds in mice, *Med. Exp.* **9**:263-267.

Davis, W. M., and Webb, O. L., 1964, Chemoconvulsive thresholds in mice of differing audioconvulsive susceptibilities, *Experientia* **20**:291.

Davis, W. M., Babbini, M., Pong, S. F., King, W. T., and White, C. L., 1974, Motility of mice after amphetamine: Effects of strain, aggregation and illumination, *Pharmacol. Biochem. Behav.* **2**:803-809.

Deckard, B. S., Lieff, B., Schlesinger, K., and DeFries, J. C., 1976, Developmental patterns of seizure susceptibility in inbred strains of mice, *Dev. Psychobiol.* **9**:17-24.

DeFries, J. C., and Hegmann, J. P., 1970, Genetic analysis of open-field behavior, in: *Contributions to Behavior–Genetic Analysis: The Mouse as a Prototype* (G. Lindzey and D. D. Thiessen, eds.), pp. 23-56, Appleton-Century-Crofts, New York.

DeLuca, D. C., Murphree, O. D., and Angel, C., 1974, Biochemistry of nervous dogs, *Pavlov. J. Biol. Sci.* **9**:139-148.

Drewek, K. J., and Broadhurst, P. L., 1978, Ethanol preference in strains of rats selectively bred for behavior, *J. Stud. Alcohol,* submitted.

Driscoll, P., 1976, Nicotine-like behavioral effect after small dose of mecamylamine in Roman high-avoidance rats, *Psychopharmacologia* **46**:119-121.

Dudek, B. C., 1977, Acetaldehyde as a psychopharmacological agent: Task specificity of genotypic differences, *Behav. Genet.* **7**:56-57 (abstract).

Dykman, R. A., Murphree, O. D., and Peters, J. E., 1969, Like begets like: Behavioral tests, classical autonomic and motor conditioning, and operant conditioning in two strains of Pointer dogs, *Ann. N. Y. Acad. Sci.* **159**:976-1007.

Eaves, L. J., and Brumpton, R. J., 1972, Factors of covariation in *Nicotiana rustica,* *Heredity* **29**:151-175.

Eleftheriou, B. E., 1974, Genetic analysis of hypothalamic retention of [³H] corticosterone in two inbred strains of mice, *Brain Res.* **66**:77-82.

Eleftheriou, B. E., 1975*a*, Hormones and behavior: A genetic approach, in: *Hormonal Correlates of Behavior,* Vol. 2, *An Organismic Approach* (B. E. Eleftheriou and R. L. Sprott, eds.), pp. 447-467, Plenum Press, New York.

Eleftheriou, B. E. (ed.), 1975*b*, *Psychopharmacogenetics,* Plenum Press, New York.

Eleftheriou, B. E., 1975*c*, Psychopharmacogenetics: An integrative approach to the study of genes, drugs and behavior, in *Psychopharmacogenetics* (B. E. Eleftheriou, ed.), pp. 1-10, Plenum Press, New York.

Eleftheriou, B. E., and Bailey, D. W., 1972*a*, A gene controlling plasma serotonin levels in mice, *J. Endocrinol.* **55**:225-226.

Eleftheriou, B. E., and Bailey, D. W., 1972*b*, Genetic analysis of plasma corticosterone levels in two inbred strains of mice, *J. Endocrinol.* **55**:415-420.

Eleftheriou, B. E., and Elias, P. K., 1975, Recombinant inbred strains: A novel genetic approach for psychopharmacogeneticists, in: *Psychopharmacogenetics* (B. E. Eleftheriou, ed.), pp. 43-71, Plenum Press, New York.

Eleftheriou, B. E., and Kristal, M. B., 1974, A gene controlling bell- and photically-induced ovulation in mice, *J. Reprod. Fertil.* **38**:41-47.

Eleftheriou, B. E., Bailey, D. W., and Denenberg, V. H., 1974, Genetic analysis of fighting behavior in mice, *Physiol. Behav.* **13**:773-777.

Eleftheriou, B. E., Elias, M. F., Cherry, M., and Lucas, L., 1976, Relationships of wheel running activity to post-wheel running plasma testosterone and corticosterone levels: A behavior–genetic analysis, *Physiol. Behav.* **16**:431-438.

Elias, M. F., and Eleftheriou, B. E., 1975*a*, A behavior-genetic investigation of induction and eduction times for halothane anesthesia, *Behav. Res. Meth. Instrum.* **7**:7-10.

Elias, M. F., and Eleftheriou, B. E., 1975*b*, Genetic analysis of simple water escape behavior: Test of a major-gene hypothesis, *Physiol. Behav.* **15**:737-740.

Elias, M. F., and Pentz, C. A., 1975, The role of genotype in behavioral responses in anesthetics, in: *Psychopharmacogenetics* (B. E. Eleftheriou, ed.), pp. 229-321, Plenum Press, New York.

Elias, M. F., and Simmerman, S. J., 1971, Proactive and retroactive effects of diethyl ether on spatial discrimination learning in inbred mouse strains DBA/2J and C57BL/6J, *Psychon. Sci.* **22**:229-301.

Ellinwood, E. H., Jr., and Kilbey, M. M., 1975, Species differences in response to amphetamine, in: *Psychopharmacogenetics* (B. E. Eleftheriou, ed.), pp. 223-375, Plenum Press, New York.

Eriksson, C. J. P., 1973, Ethanol and acetaldehyde metabolism in rat strains genetically selected for their ethanol preference, *Biochem. Pharmacol.* **22**:2283-2292.

Eriksson, K., 1965, Genetiska faktorer i försöksdjurs alkoholpreferens (On hereditary factors in voluntary alcohol consumption), *Alkoholpolitik* **28**:114-118, 152-154.

Eriksson, K., 1968a, En biologisk utredning över alkoholismens etiologi med djurexperiment (A biological approach to the etiology of alcoholism through experimentation), *Alkoholpolitik* **31**:111-117.

Eriksson, K., 1968b, Genetic selection for voluntary alcohol consumption in the albino rat, *Science* **159**:739-741.

Eriksson, K., 1968c, Periman ja ympariston ossuus alkoholin nauttimista saatelevina tekijoina koe-elaimilla suoritettujen tutkimusten perusteela (The genotype and phenotype as factors regulating alcohol consumption in laboratory animals), *Alkoholikysymys* **36**:3-9.

Eriksson, K., 1969a, The estimation of heritability for the self-selection of alcohol in the albino rat, *Ann. Med. Exp. Fenn.* **47**:172-174.

Eriksson, K., 1969b, Factors affecting voluntary alcohol consumption in the albino rat, *Ann. Zool. Fennici* **6**:227-265.

Eriksson, K., 1971a, Inheritance of behaviour towards alcohol in normal and motivated choice situation in mice, *Ann. Zool. Fennici* **8**:400-405.

Eriksson, K., 1971b, Rat strains specially selected for their voluntary alcohol consumption, *Ann. Med. Exp. Biol. Fenn.* **49**:67-72.

Eriksson, K., 1972a, Alcohol consumption and blood alcohol in rat strains selected for their behavior towards alcohol, in: *International Symposium Biological Aspects of Alcohol Consumption, 27-29 September 1971, Helsinki,* Vol. 20 (O. Forsander and K. Eriksson, eds.), pp. 121-125, The Finnish Foundation for Alcohol Studies, Helsinki.

Eriksson, K., 1972b, Behavioral and physiological differences among rat strains specially selected for their alcohol consumption, *Ann. N. Y. Acad. Sci* **197**:32-41.

Eriksson, K., 1972c, Rat strains genetically selected for their behavior towards alcohol, *Scand. J. Clin. Lab. Invest.* **29**:53.

Eriksson, K., 1974, Genetic aspects of alcohol drinking behaviour, *Int. J. Neurol.* **9**:125-133.

Eriksson, K., 1975, Alcohol imbibition and behavior: A comparative genetic approach, in: *Psychopharmacogenetics* (B. E. Eleftheriou, ed.), pp. 127-168, Plenum Press, New York.

Eriksson, K., and Kiianmaa, K., 1971, Genetic analysis of susceptibility to morphine addiction in inbred mice, *Ann. Med. Exp. Biol. Fenn.* **49**:73-78.

Eriksson, K., and Malmström, K. K., 1967, Sex differences in consumption and elimination of alcohol in albino rats, *Ann. Med. Exp. Fenn.* **45**:389-392.

Eriksson, K., and Närhi, M., 1973, Specially selected rat strains as a model of alcoholism, in: *The Laboratory Animal in Drug Testing* (A. Spiegel, ed.), pp. 163-171, Fischer Verlag, Stuttgart.

Eriksson, K., and Pikkarainen, P. H., 1968, Differences between the sexes in voluntary alcohol consumption and liver ADH-activity in inbred strains of mice, *Metabolism* **17**:1037-1042.

Eriksson, K., and Pikkarainen, P. H., 1970, Strain and sex differences in voluntary alcohol consumption, liver ADH activity and aldehyde oxidizing capacity in inbred strains of mice, *Jpn. J. Stud. Alcohol* **5**:1-7.

Erwin, V. G., Heston, W. D. W., McClearn, G., and Deitrich, R. A., 1976, Effect of hypnotics on mice genetically selected for sensitivity to ethanol, *Pharmacol. Biochem. Behav.* **4**:679-683.

Eysenck, H. J., 1957, *The Dynamics of Anxiety and Hysteria: An Experimental Application of Modern Learning Theory to Psychiatry,* Routledge and Kegan Paul, London.

Eysenck, H. J., and Broadhurst, P. L., 1964, Experiments with animals: Introduction, in: *Experiments in Motivation* (H. J. Eysenck, ed.), pp. 285-291, Pergamon Press, Oxford.

Falconer, D. S., 1960, *Introduction to Quantitative Genetics,* Oliver and Boyd, Edinburgh.

Festing, M., and Staats, J., 1973, Standardized nomenclature for inbred strains of rats, fourth listing, *Transplantation* **16**:221-245.

Finger, F. W., 1969, Estrus and general activity in the rat, *J. Comp. Physiol. Psychol.* **68**: 461-466.

Fleming, J. C., and Broadhurst, P. L., 1975, The effects of nicotine on two-way avoidance conditioning in bi-directionally selected strains of rats, *Psychopharmacologia* **42**:147-152.

Flood, J. F., Rosenzweig, M. R., Bennett, E. L., and Orme, A. E., 1974, Comparison of the effects of anisomycin on memory across six strains of mice, *Behav. Biol.* **10**:147-160.

Forsander, O. A., and Eriksson, C. J. P., 1972, Metabolic characteristics of rat strains consuming different amounts of alcohol, in: *International Symposium on the Biological Aspects of Alcohol Consumption, 27-29 September 1971,* Vol. 20 (O. A. Forsander and K. Eriksson, eds.), pp. 43-49, The Finnish Foundation for Alcohol Studies, Helsinki.

Fulker, D. W., 1970, Maternal buffering of rodent genotypic responses to stress: A complex genotype-environment interaction, *Behav. Genet.* **1**:119-124.

Fulker, D. W., Wilcock, J., and Broadhurst, P. L., 1972, Studies in genotype-environment interaction. I. Methodology and preliminary multivariate analysis of a diallel cross of eight strains of rat, *Behav. Genet.* **2**:261-287.

Fuller, J. L., 1964, Measurement of alcohol preference in genetic experiments, *J. Comp. Physiol. Psychol.* **57**:85-88.

Fuller, J. L., 1966, Variation in effects of chlorpromazine in three strains of mice, *Psychopharmacologia* **8**:408-414.

Fuller, J. L., 1970*a*, Pharmacogenetics, in: *Principles of Psychopharmacology: A Textbook for Physicians, Medical Students and Behavioral Scientists* (W. G. Clark and J. del Giudice, eds.), pp. 337-342, Academic Press, New York.

Fuller, J. L., 1970*b*, Strain differences in the effects of chlorpormazine and chlordiazepoxide upon active and passive avoidance in mice, *Psychopharmacologia* **16**:261-271.

Fuller, J. L., and Church, A. C., 1977, Voluntary ethanol consumption by mice selected for differing sleep times following acute ethanol administration, *Behav. Genet.* **7**:59 (abstract).

Fuller, J. L., and Clark, L. D., 1966, Genetic and treatment factors modifying the postisolation syndrome in dogs, *J. Comp. Physiol. Psychol.* **61**:251-257.

Fuller, J. L., and Collins, R. L., 1972, Ethanol consumption and preference in mice: A genetic analysis, *Ann. N. Y. Acad. Sci.* **197**:42-48.

Fuller, J. L., and Hansult, C. D., 1975, Genes and drugs as behavior modifying agents, in: *Psychopharmacogenetics* (B. E. Eleftheriou, ed.), pp. 11-18, Plenum Press, New York.

Garg, M., 1968, The effect of nicotine on rearing in two strains of rats, *Life Sci.* **7**:421-429.

Garg, M., 1969*a*, The effects of nicotine on two different types of learning, *Psychopharmacologia* **15**:408-414.

Garg, M., 1969*b*, The effects of some central nervous system stimulant and depressant drugs on rearing activity in rats, *Psychopharmacologia* 14:150-156.

Garg, M., 1969*c*, Variation in effects of nicotine in four strains of rats, *Psychopharmacologia* 14:432-438.

Garg, M., 1970, Combined effect of drug and drive on the consolidation process, *Psychopharmacologia* 18:172-179.

Garg, M., and Holland, H. C., 1967, Consolidation and maze learning: A comparison of several post-trial treatments, *Life Sci.* 6:1987-1997.

Garg, M., and Holland, H.C., 1968*a*, Consolidation and maze learning: A further study of post-trial injections of a stimulant drug (nicotine), *Int. J. Neuropharmacol.* 7:55-59.

Garg, M., and Holland, H. C., 1968*b*, Consolidation and maze learning: The effects of post-trial injections of a depressant drug (pentobarbital sodium), *Psychopharmacologia* 12: 127-132.

Garg, M., and Holland, H. C., 1968*c*, Consolidation and maze learning: The effects of post-trial injections of a stimulant drug (picrotoxin), *Psychopharmacologia* 12:96-103.

Garg, M., and Holland, H. C., 1969, Consolidation and maze learning: A study of some strain/drug interactions, *Psychopharmacologia* 14:426-431.

Gay, P. E., and Leaf, R. C., 1976, Rat strain differences in pilocarpine-induced mouse killing, *Physiol. Psychol.* 4:28-32.

Gebhart, G. F., and Mitchell, C. L., 1973, Strain differences in the analgesic response to morphine as measured on the hot plate, *Arch. Int. Pharmacodyn. Ther.* 201:128-140.

Ginsburg, B. E., Becker, R. E., Trattner, A., Dutson, J., and Bareggi, S. R., 1976, Genetic variation in drug response in hybrid dogs: A possible model for the hyperkinetic syndrome, *Behav. Genet.* 6:107 (abstract).

Ginsburg, B. E., Yanai, J., and Hedrick, B., 1977, Nutritionally mediated effects of alcohol administered to pregnant and lactating mice on the behavior of their offspring, *Behav. Genet.* 7:61-62 (abstract).

Goldstein, D. B., 1973, Inherited differences in intensity of alcohol withdrawal reactions in mice, *Nature (London)* 245:154-156.

Goldstein, D. B., and Kakihana, R., 1974, Alcohol withdrawal reactions and reserpine effects in inbred strains of mice, *Life Sci.* 15:415-425.

Goldstein, D. B., and Kakihana, R., 1975, Alcohol withdrawal reactions in mouse strains selectively bred for long or short sleep times, *Life Sci.* 17:981-986.

Goodrick, C. L., 1972, End bottle preferences of inbred mice during alcohol preference and fluid intake multiple-bottle test procedures, *Psychon. Sci.* 28:185-187.

Gray, J. A., 1964, *Pavlov's Typology: Recent Theoretical and Experimental Developments from the Laboratory of B. M. Teplov,* Pergamon Press, Oxford.

Green, E. L., and Meier, H., 1965, Use of laboratory animals for the analysis of genetic influences upon drug toxicity, *Ann. N. Y. Acad. Sci.* 123:295-304.

Greenough, W. T., and McGaugh, J. L., 1965, The effect of strychnine sulphate on learning as a function of time of administration, *Psychopharmacologia* 8:290-294.

Gregory, K., 1967, A note on the action of methyl pentynol carbamate in strains of rats bred for differential conditioning ability, *Psychopharmacologia* 11:317-319.

Gregory, K., 1968*a*, The action of the drug Prenylamine (segontin) on exploratory activity and aversive learning in a selected strain of rats, *Psychopharmacologia* 13:22-28.

Gregory, K., 1968*b*, The action of the drug prenylamine (segontin) on exploratory activity in strains of rats selectively bred for differences in emotionality, *Psychopharmacologia* 13: 29-34.

Gregory, K., Gupta, B. D., and Holland, H. C., 1967, The effects of drugs on activity in two strains of rats selectively bred for high and low emotionality, *Life Sci.* **6**:981-988.

Gunn, J. A., and Gurd, M. R., 1940, The action of some amines related to adrenaline cyclohexylalkylamines, *J. Physiol.* **97**:453-470.

Gupta, B. D., and Gregory, K., 1967, The effect of drugs and their combinations on the rearing response in two strains of rats, *Psychopharmacologia* **11**:365-371.

Gupta, B. D., and Holland, H. C., 1969*a*, An examination of the effects of stimulant and depressant drugs on escape/avoidance conditioning in strains of rats selectively bred for emotionality/non-emotionality, *Psychopharmacologia* **14**:95-105.

Gupta, B. D., and Holland, H. C., 1969*b*, An examination of the effects of stimulant and depressant drugs on escape/avoidance conditioning in strains of rats selectively bred for emotionality/non-emotionality: Intertrial activity, *Int. J. Neuropharmacol* **8**:227-234.

Gupta, B.D., and Holland, H.C., 1972, Emotion as a determinant of the effects of drugs and their combination on different components of behaviour in rats, *Neuropharmacology* **11**:31-38.

Gut, I., and Becker, B. A., 1975, Heredity of hexobarbital sleeping time and efficiency of drug metabolism in Wistar and Sprague–Dawley rats, *Arch. Toxicol.* **34**:61-70.

Hall, C. S., 1934, Emotional behavior in the rat: I. Defecation and urination as measures of individual differences in emotionality, *J. Comp. Psychol.* **18**:385-403.

Hatchell, P. C., and Collins, A. C., 1977, Influences of genotype and sex on behavioral tolerance to nicotine in mice, *Pharmacol. Biochem. Behav.* **6**:25-30.

Heinze, W. J., 1974, Genotype influences on ether-induced retrograde amnesia in rats, *Behav. Biol.* **11**:109-114.

Henderson, N. D., 1968, Genetic analysis of acquisition and retention of conditioned fear in mice, *J. Comp. Physiol. Psychol.* **65**:325-329.

Henry, K. R., and Schlesinger, K., 1967, Effects of the albino and dilute loci on mouse behavior, *J. Comp. Physiol. Psychol.* **63**:320-323.

Heston, W. D. W., Anderson, S. M., Erwin, V. G., and McClearn, G. E., 1973, A comparison of the actions of various hypnotics on mice selectively bred for sensitivity to ethanol, *Behav. Genet.* **3**:402-403 (abstract).

Heston, W. D. W., Erwin, V. G., Anderson, S. M., and Robbins, H., 1974, A comparison of the effects of alcohol on mice selectively bred for differences in ethanol sleep-time, *Life Sci.* **14**:365-370.

Hillman, M. G., and Schneider, C. W., 1975, Voluntary selection and tolerance to 1, 2 propanediol (propylene glycol) by high and low ethanol-selecting mouse strains, *J. Comp. Physiol. Psychol.* **88**:773-777.

Ho, A. K. S., Tsai, C. S., and Kissin, B., 1975, Neurochemical correlates of alcohol preference in inbred strains of mice, *Pharmacol. Biochem. Behav.* **3**:1073-1076.

Holland, H. C., and Gupta, B. D., 1966, The effects of different doses of methylpentynol on escape-avoidance conditioning in two strains of rats selectively bred for high and low "emotionality," *Psychopharmacologia* **9**:419-425.

Holland, H. C., and Gupta, B. D., 1967, Effects of drugs on the rearing response in emotionally reactive and non-reactive rats, *Act. Nerv. Super.* **9**:134-136.

Horowitz, G. P., 1976, Morphine self administration by inbred mice: A preliminary report, *Behav. Genet.* **6**:109-110 (abstract).

Huff, S. D., 1962, A genetically controlled response to the drug chlorpromazine, *Genetics* **47**:962 (abstract).

Isaeva, I. I., and Krasuskii, V. K., 1961, K voprosu o nasledovanii reaktsii tsentral'noi nervnoi sistemy sobak na vvedenie kofeina (On the problem of inheritance of the central nervous system's reaction to the injection of caffeine in dogs), *Dokl. Akad. Nauk SSSR* **141**:248-251 [*Psychol. Abstr.* 1962, **36**:5, 5DK481 (abstract)].

Jinks, J. L., and Broadhurst, P. L., 1974, How to analyse the inheritance of behaviour in animals—the biometrical approach, in: *The Genetics of Behaviour* (J. H. F. van Abeelen, ed.), pp. 1-41, North Holland Publishing Co., Amsterdam.

Jinks, J. L., and Pooni, H. S., 1976, Predicting the properties of recombinant inbred lines derived by single seed descent, *Heredity* 36:253-266.

Joffe, J. M., Najman, J., and Nettleton, N., 1976, Environmental effects on alcohol selection by mice, *Nature (London)* 262:725-762.

Jones, R. M., 1965, Analysis of variance of the half diallel table, *Heredity* 20:117-121.

Kahn, A. J., 1974, Changes in ethanol consumption by C3H and CF1 mice with age, *J. Stud. Alcohol* 36:1107-1123.

Kakihana, R., 1976, Adrenocortical function in mice selectively bred for different sensitivity to ethanol, *Life Sci.* 18:1131-1138.

Kakihana, R., and Moore, J., 1977, Ethanol-induced hypo- and hyperthermia in inbred strains of mice and mice selectively bred for ethanol sensitivity, *Behav. Genet.* 7:76 (abstract).

Kalow, W., 1962, *Pharmacogenetics: Heredity and the Response to Drugs,* Saunders, Philadelphia.

Karczmar, A. G., and Scudder, C. L., 1969, Learning and effects of drugs on learning of related mice genera and strains, in: *Neurophysiological and Behavioral Aspects of Psychotropic Drugs* (A. G. Karczmar and W. P. Koella, eds.), pp. 133-160, C. C. Thomas, Springfield, Illinois.

Keeler, C. E., and Fromm, E., 1965, Genes, drugs and behavior in foxes, *J. Hered.* 56:288-291.

Keeler, C. E., and King, H. D., 1941, Multiple effects of coat-color genes in the rat, with special reference to the "marks of domestication," *Anat. Rec.* 81:48-49 (abstract).

Keehn, J. D., 1972, Effects of trihexphenidyl on schedule-induced alcohol drinking by rats, *Psychon. Sci.* 29:20-22.

Keenan, A., and Johnson, F. N., 1972, Development of behavioral tolerance to nicotine in the rat, *Experientia* 28:428-429.

Kiianmaa, K., 1975, Evidence for involvement of noradrenaline and against 5-hydroxytryptamine neurons in alcohol consumption by rats, in: *The Effects of Centrally Active Drugs on Voluntary Alcohol Consumption* (J. D. Sinclair and K. Kiianmaa, eds.), pp. 73-84, The Finnish Foundation for Alcohol Studies, Helsinki.

Kitahama, K., and Valatx, J.-L., 1975, Action de l'α-methyl-dopa sur les rythmes veille-sommeil des souris C57BR et C57BL/6, *Psychopharmacologia* 45:189-196.

Kitahama, K., Valatx, J.-L., and Jouvet, M., 1975, Action differente de l'α-methyl-DOPA sur le sommeil et l'acquisition d'un labyrinthe chez deux souches consanguines de souris, *C. R. Acad. Sci.* 280:471-474.

Kitahama, K., Valatx, J.-L., and Jouvet, M., 1976, Apprentissage d'un labyrinthe en y chez deux souches de souris. Effets de la privation instrumentale et pharmacologique du sommeil, *Brain Res.* 108:75-86.

Klein, T. W., 1977, Genetic analysis using recombinant inbred strains and histocompatibility lines, *Behav. Genet.* 7:71-72 (abstract).

Koivula, T., and Lindros, K. O., 1975, Effects of long-term ethanol treatment on aldehyde and alcohol dehydrogenase activities in rat liver, *Biochem. Pharmacol.* 24:1937-1942.

Koivula, T., Koivusalo, M., and Lindros, K. O., 1975, Liver aldehyde and alcohol dehydrogenase activities in rat strains genetically selected for their ethanol preference, *Biochem. Pharmacol.* 24:1807-1811.

Komura, S., 1974, Effects of ethyleneglycol dinitrate and related compounds on ethanol preference and ethanol metabolism, *Acta Pharmacol. Toxicol.* 35:145-154.

Komura, S., Ueda, M., and Kobayashi, T., 1972, Effects of foster nursing on alcohol selection in inbred strains of mice, *Q. J. Stud. Alcohol* 33:494-503.

Krivanek, J., and McGaugh, J. L., 1968, Fffects of pentylenetetrazol on memory storage in mice, *Psychopharmacologia* **12**:303-321.

Kumar, R., and Stolerman, I. P., 1973, Morphine dependent behaviour in rats: Some clinical implications, *Psychol. Med.* **3**:225-237.

Lagerspetz, K. Y. H., and Lagerspetz, K. M. J., 1971, Amphetamine toxicity in genetically aggressive and non-aggressive mice, *J. Pharm. Pharmacol.* **23**:542-543.

Lapin, I. P., 1967, Simple pharmacological procedures to differentiate anti-depressants and cholinolytics in mice and rats, *Psychopharmacologia* **11**:79-87.

Lapin, I. P., 1974, Behavioural effects of psychoactive drugs influencing the metabolism of brain monoamines in mice of different strains, in: *Genetics of Behaviour* (J. H. F. van Abeelen, ed.), pp. 417-432, North Holland Publishing Co., Amsterdam.

Lapin, I. P., 1975, Effects of apomorphine in mice of different strains, in: *Psychopharmacogenetics* (B. E. Eleftheriou, ed.), pp. 19-33, Plenum Press, New York.

Lát, J., and Gollová, E., 1964, Drug-induced increase of central nervous excitability and the emergence of spontaneous stereotyped reactions, *Act. Nerv. Super.* **6**(2):200-201.

Lát, J., and Gollová-Hémon, E., 1969, Permanent effects of nutritional and endocrinological intervention in early ontogeny on the level of nonspecific excitability and on lability (emotionality), *Ann. N. Y. Acad. Sci.* **159**:710-720.

Lester, D., 1966, Self-selection of alcohol by animals, human variation and the etiology of alcoholism: A critical review, *Q. J. Stud. Alcohol* **27**:395-458.

Lester, D., and Freed, E. X., 1972, A rat model of alcoholism? *Ann. N. Y. Acad. Sci.* **197**: 54-59.

Lucas, L. A., and Eleftheriou, B. E., 1975, Association between plasma testosterone and aggressiveness: A genetic analysis, *Behav. Genet.* **5**:100 (abstract).

Lucas, L. A., and Scott, J. P., 1977, Hyperactivity in two dog breeds and their hybrids, *Behav. Genet.* **7**:74-75 (abstract).

Lush, I. E., 1975a, A comparison of the effect of mescaline on activity and emotional defaecation in seven strains of mice, *Br. J. Pharmacol.* **55**:133-139.

Lush, I. E., 1975b, A relationship between hexobarbitone sleeping time and susceptibility to mescaline in mice from different strains, *Psychopharmacologia* **43**:259-260.

MacInnes, J. W., and Damjanovich, R. P., 1973, Analysis of several parameters influencing ethanol sleep-time in inbred and selectively bred mice, *Behav. Genet.* **3**:408 (abstract).

MacInnes, J. W., and Uphouse, L. L., 1973, Effects of alcohol on acquisition and retention of passive-avoidance conditioning in different mouse strains, *J. Comp. Physiol. Psychol.* **84**:398-402.

Mackintosh, J. H., 1962, Effect of strain and group size on the response of mice to 'seconal' anaesthesia, *Nature (London)* **194**:1034.

Mandel, P., Ebel, A., Mack, G., and Kempf, E., 1974, Neurochemical correlates of behaviour in mouse strains, in: *Genetics of Behaviour* (J. H. F. van Abeelen, ed.), pp. 397-415, North Holland Publishing Co., Amsterdam.

Mardones, J., 1960, Experimentally induced changes in the free selection of ethanol, *Int. Rev. Neurobiol.* **2**:41-76.

Mardones, J., 1968, Pharmacogénétique de l'alcoolisme, *Actual. Pharmacol.* **21**:1-13.

Mardones, R. J., Segovia, M. N., and Hederra, D. A., 1950, Herencia del alcoholismo en ratas. I. Comportamiento de la primera generación de ratas bebedoras, colocadas en dieta carenciada en factor N (The inheritance of alcoholism in rats: I. Behavior of the first generation of addicted rats reared on a diet lacking in factor N), *Bol. Soc. Biol. Santiago* **7**: 61-62 [*Suppl. Rev. Med. Aliment. Santiago* 1950, **9**].

Mardones, R. J., Segovia, M. N., and Hederra, D. A., 1953, Heredity of experimental alcohol preference in rats. II. Coefficient of heredity, *Q. J. Stud. Alcohol* **14**:1-2.

Marselos, M., Eriksson, K., and Hänninen, O., 1975, Aldehyde dehydrogenase inducibility and ethanol preference in rats, *Med. Biol.* **53**:224-230.

Martin, L. K., and Powell, B. J., 1970, Role of drug effects and UCS intensity in avoidance acquisition of the Maudsley MNR and MR strains, *Psychon. Sci.* **18**:44-51.

Masur, J., and Benedito, M. A. C., 1974*a*, Genetic selection of winner and loser rats in a competitive situation, *Nature (London)* **249**:284.

Masur, J., and Benedito, M. A. C., 1974*b*, Inversion by apomorphine of the tendency of female rats to be defeated by males when competing for food in a straight runway, *Behav. Biol.* **10**:527-531.

Masur, J., Maroni, J. B., and Benedito, M. A. C., 1975, Genetically selected winner and loser rats in the tunnel competition: Influence of apomorphine and dopa, *Behav. Biol.* **14**:21-30.

Mather, K., 1946, The genetical requirements of bio-assays with higher organisms, *Analyst* **71**:407-411.

Mather, K., and Jinks, J. L., 1971, *Biometrical Genetics: The Study of Continuous Variation,* 2nd ed., Chapman and Hall, London.

Maxson, S. C., Sze, P. Y., and Cowen, J. S., 1975, Pharmacogenetics of the sensory induction of susceptibility to audiogenic seizures in two strains of mice, *Behav. Genet.* **5**:102 (abstract).

McBryde, W. O., and Murphree, O. D., 1974, The rehabilitation of genetically nervous dogs, *Pavlov. J. Biol. Sci.* **9**:76-84.

McClearn, G. E., 1972*a*, The genetics of alcohol preference, in: *International Symposium on the Biological Aspects of Alcohol Consumption, 27-29 September, 1971,* Vol. 20 (O. Forsander and K. Eriksson, eds.), pp. 113-119, The Finnish Foundation for Alcohol Studies, Helsinki.

McClearn, G. E., 1972*b*, Genetics as a tool in alcohol research, *Ann. N. Y. Acad. Sci.* **197**:26-31.

McClearn, G. E., 1973, The genetic aspects of alcoholism, in: *Alcoholism: Progress in Research and Treatment* (P. G. Bourne and R. Fox, eds.), pp. 337-358, Academic Press, New York.

McClearn, G. E., and Kakihana, R., 1973, Selective breeding for ethanol sensitivity in mice, *Behav. Genet.* **3**:409-410 (abstract).

McClearn, G. E., and Rodgers, D. A., 1959, Differences in alcohol preferences among inbred strains of mice, *Q. J. Stud. Alcohol.* **20**:691-695.

McClearn, G. E., and Rodgers, D. A., 1961, Genetic factors in alcohol preference of laboratory mice, *J. Comp. Physiol. Psychol.* **54**:116-119.

McClearn, G. E., and Shern, D. L., 1975, The effects of intraperitoneal ethanol injections on the locomotor activity of five inbred strains of mice, *Behav. Genet.* **5**:103 (abstract).

McGaugh, J. L., 1961, Facilitative and disruptive effects of strychnine sulphate on maze learning, *Psychol. Rep.* **8**:99-104.

McGaugh, J. L., 1973, Drug facilitation of learning and memory, *Ann. Rev. Pharmacol.* **13**:229-241.

McGaugh, J. L., and Herz, M. J., 1972, *Memory Consolidation,* Albion, San Francisco.

McGaugh, J. L., and Petrinovich, L., 1959, The effect of strychnine sulphate on maze-learning, *Am. J. Psychol.* **72**:99-102.

McGaugh, J. L., and Thomson, C. W., 1962, Facilitation of discrimination learning with strychnine sulphate, *Psychopharmacologia,* **3**:166-172.

McGaugh, J. L., Westbrook, W., and Burt, G., 1961, Strain differences in the facilitative effects of 5-7 Diphenyl-1-3-Diazadamantan-6-ol (1757 I.S.) on maze learning, *J. Comp. Physiol. Psychol.* **54**:502-505.

McGaugh, J. L., Westbrook, W. H., and Thomson, C. W., 1962a, Facilitation of maze learning with post-trial injections of 5-7-Diphenyl-1-3-Diazadamantan-6-ol (1757 I.S.), *J. Comp. Physiol. Psychol.* **55**:710-713.

McGaugh, J. L., Thomson, C. W., Westbrook, W. H., and Hudspeth, W. J., 1962b, A further study of learning facilitation with strychnine sulphate, *Psychopharmacologia* **3**:352-360.

McLaren, A., and Michie, D., 1956, Variability of response in experimental animals: A comparison of the reactions of inbred, F_1 hybrid and random bred mice to a narcotic drug, *J. Genet.* **54**:440-455.

Meade, R., Amit, Z., Pachter, W., and Corcoran, M. E., 1973, Differences in oral intake of morphine by two strains of rats, *Res. Comm. Chem. Pathol. Pharmacol.* **6**:1105-1108.

Meier, G. W., Hatfield, J. L., and Foshee, D. P., 1963, Genetic and behavioural aspects of pharmacologically induced arousal, *Psychopharmacologia* **4**:81-90.

Meier, H., 1963, *Experimental Pharmacogenetics. Physiopathology of Heredity and Pharmacologic Responses,* Academic Press, New York.

Melchior, C. L., and Myers, R. D., 1976, Genetic differences in ethanol drinking of the rat following injection of 6-OHDA, 5,6-DHT or 5,7-DHT into the cerebral ventricles, *Pharmacol. Biochem. Behav.* **5**:63-72.

Messeri, P., Eleftheriou, E., and Oliverio, A., 1975, Dominance behavior: A phylogenetic analysis in the mouse, *Physiol. Behav.* **14**:53-58.

Michelson, M. J., 1974, Some aspects of evolutionary pharmacology, *Biochem. Pharmacol.* **23**:2211-2244.

Moisset, B., 1977, Genetic analysis of cerebral norepinephrine uptake and open-field activity, *Behav. Genet.* **7**:78-79 (abstract).

Moisset, B., and Welch, B. L., 1973, Effects of *d*-amphetamine upon open field behaviour in two inbred strains of mice, *Experientia* **29**:625-626.

Morrison, C. F., 1969, The effects of nicotine on punished behaviour, *Psychopharmacologia* **14**:221-232.

Morrison, C. F., and Lee, P. N., 1968, A comparison of the effects of nicotine and physostigmine on a measure of activity in the rat, *Psychopharmacologia* **13**:210-221.

Morrison, C. F., and Stephenson, J. A., 1973, Effects of stimulants on observed behaviour of rats on six operant schedules, *Neuropharmacology* **12**:297-310.

Müller-Calgan, H., and Schorscher, E., 1973, The significance of exogenous and endogenous factors in the hereditary differences in learning ability of rats, in: *Memory and Transfer of Information* (H. P. Zippel, ed.), pp. 65-85, Plenum Press, New York.

Müller-Calgan, H., Becker, K. H., Enenkel, H. J., Schliep, H. J., and Wild, A. J. N., 1973, The reactivity of Wistar rats highly selected for good and bad learning, observed in various physiological and pharmacological test models: 1st communication, in: *Memory and Transfer of Information* (H. P. Zippel, ed.), pp. 87-125, Plenum Press, New York.

Murphree, O. D., 1972, Reduction of anxiety in genetically timid dogs: Drug-induced schizokinesis and autokinesis, *Cond. Reflex* **7**:170-176.

Murphree, O. D., 1973, Inheritance of human aversion and inactivity in two strains of the pointer dog, *Biol. Psychiat.* **7**:23-29.

Murphree, O. D., and Dykman, R. A., 1965, Litter patterns in the offspring of nervous and stable dogs. I. Behavioral tests, *J. Nerv. Ment. Dis.* **141**:321-332.

Murphree, O. D., and Newton, J. E. O., 1971, Crossbreeding and special handling of genetically nervous dogs, *Cond. Reflex* **6**:129-136.

Murphree, O. D., Dykman, R. A., and Peters, J. E., 1967a, Genetically-determined abnormal behavior in dogs: Results of behavioral test, *Cond. Reflex* **2**:199-205.

Murphree, O. D., Dykman, R. A., and Peters, J. E., 1967b, Operant conditioning of two strains of the pointer dog, *Psychophysiology* **3**:414-417.

Murphree, O. D., Peters, J. E., and Dykman, R. A., 1969, Behavioral comparisons of nervous, stable, and crossbred pointers at ages 2, 3, 6, 9, and 12 months, *Cond. Reflex* **4**:20-23.

Murphree, O. D., Angel, C., and DeLuca, D. C., 1974*a*, Limits of therapeutic change: Specificity of behavior modification in genetically nervous dogs, *Biol. Psychiat.* **9**:99-101.

Murphree, O. D., DeLuca, D. C., and Angel, C., 1974*b*, Psychopharmacologic facilitation of operant conditioning of genetically nervous catahoula and pointer dogs, *Pavlov. J. Biol. Sci.* **9**:17-24.

Myers, R. D., and Eriksson, K., 1968, Ethyl alcohol consumption: Valid measurement in albino rats, *Science* **161**:76-77.

Myers, R. D., and Holman, R. B., 1966, A procedure for eliminating position habit in preference-aversion tests for ethanol and other fluids, *Psychonom. Sci.* **6**:235-236.

Myers, R. D., and Melchior, C. L., 1975, Dietary tryptophan and the selection of ethyl alcohol in different strains of rats, *Psychopharmacologia* **42**:109-115.

Nachman, M., 1959, The inheritance of saccharin preference, *J. Comp. Physiol. Psychol.* **52**:451-457.

Nachman, M., Lester, D., and Le Magnen, J., 1970, Alcohol aversion in the rat: Behavioral assessment of noxious drug effects, *Science* **168**:1244-1245.

Nachman, M., Larue, C., and Le Magnen, J., 1971, The role of olfactory and orosensory factors in the alcohol preference of inbred strains of mice, *Physiol. Behav.* **6**:53-60.

Newton, J. E. O., Chapin, J. L., and Murphree, O. D., 1976, Correlations of normality and nervousness with cardiovascular functions in pointer dogs, *Pavlov. J. Biol. Sci.* **11**:105-120.

Nichols, J. R., 1962, Addiction-prone and addiction-resistant rats, *Am. Psychol.* **17**:398 (abstract).

Nichols, J. R., 1964, The effect of cross-fostering on addiction-prone and addiction-resistant strains of rats, *Am. Psychol.* **19**:529 (abstract).

Nichols, J. R., and Hsiao, S., 1967, Addiction liability of albino rats: Breeding for quantitative differences in morphine drinking, *Science* **157**:561-563.

Nikander, P., and Pekkanen, L., 1977, An inborn tolerance in alcohol-preferring rats. The lack of relationship between tolerance to ethanol and the brain microsomal (Na^+K^+) ATPase activity, *Psychopharmacology* **51**:219-223.

Oliverio, A., 1974*a*, Evolutionary mechanisms in behaviour: An intraspecific genetic approach, *J. Hum. Evol.* **3**:1-18.

Oliverio, A., 1974*b*, Genetic factors in the control of drug effects on the behaviour of mice, in: *Genetics of Behaviour* (J. H. F. van Abeelen, ed.), pp. 375-395, North Holland Publishing Co., Amsterdam.

Oliverio, A., and Bovet, D., 1975, Genetic and biochemical analysis of cholinergic mechanisms in behavior, in: *Cholinergic Mechanisms* (P. G. Waser, ed.), pp. 531-540, Raven Press, New York.

Oliverio, A., and Castellano, C., 1974, Genotype-dependent sensitivity and tolerance to morphine and heroin: Dissociation between opiate-induced running and analgesia in the mouse, *Psychopharmacologia* **39**:13-22.

Oliverio, A., and Castellano, C., 1975, Exploratory activity: Genetic analysis of its modification by various pharmacologic agents, in: *Psychopharmacogenetics* (B. E. Eleftheriou, ed.) pp. 99-126, Plenum Press, New York.

Oliverio, A., and Eleftheriou, B. E., 1976, Motor activity and alcohol: A genetic investigation in the mouse, *Physiol. Behav.* **16**:577-581.

Oliverio, A., Bovet-Nitti, F., and Bovet, D., 1966, Action de la scopamine et de quelque médicaments parasympatholytiques sur le conditionnement d'évitement chez la souris, *C. R. Acad. Sci.* **262**:1796-1801.

Oliverio, A., Eleftheriou, B. E., and Bailey, D. W., 1973*a*, Exploratory activity: Genetic analysis of its modification by scopolamine and amphetamine, *Physiol. Behav.* **10**:893-899.

Oliverio, A., Eleftheriou, B. E., and Bailey, D. W., 1973*b*, A gene influencing active avoidance performance in mice, *Physiol. Behav.* **11**:497-502.

Oliverio, A., Elias, M. F., Eleftheriou, B. E., and Castellano, C., 1975*a*, Maze learning: A genetic investigation in the mouse, *Psychol. Rep.* **36**:703-712.

Oliverio, A., Castellano, C., and Eleftheriou, B. E., 1975*b*, Morphine sensitivity and tolerance: A genetic investigation in the mouse, *Psychopharmacologia* **42**:219-224.

Overton, D. A., 1973, State-dependent learning produced by addicting drugs, in: *Opiate Addiction: Origins and Treatment* (S. Fisher and A. M. Freedman, eds.), pp. 61-74, Winston, Washington.

Overton, D. A., 1974, Experimental methods for the study of state dependent learning, *Fed. Proc., Am. Fed. Soc. Exp. Biol.* **33**:1800-1813.

Petrinovich. L., 1963, Facilitation of successive discrimination learning by strychnine sulphate, *Psychopharmacologia* **4**:103-113.

Petrinovich, L., 1967, Drug facilitation of learning: Strain differences, *Psychopharmacologia* **10**:375-378.

Pickett, R. A., and Collins, A. C., 1975, Use of genetic analysis to test the potential role of serotonin in alcohol preference, *Life Sci.* **17**:1291-1296.

Plotnikoff, N. P., 1960, Ataractics and strain differences in audiogenic seizures in mice, *Psychopharmacologia* **1**:429-432.

Plotnikoff, N. P., 1963*a*, Effect of psychoactive drugs on escape from audiogenic seizures, *Arch. Int. Pharmacodyn.* **145**:413-420.

Plotnikoff, N. P., 1963*b*, A neuropharmacological study of ecape from audiogenic seizures, *Colloq. Int. C.N.R.S.* **112**:429-446.

Poley, W., 1972, Alcohol-preferring and alcohol-avoiding C57BL mice, *Behav. Genet.* **2**:245-248.

Poley, W., and Mos, L., 1974, Emotionality and alcohol selection in deer mice *(Peromyscus maniculatus),* *Q. J. Stud. Alcohol.* **35**:59-65.

Poley, W., Yeudall, L. T., and Royce, J. R., 1970, Factors of emotionality related to alcohol consumption in laboratory mice, *Multivar. Behav. Res.* **5**:203-208.

Powell, B. J., 1967, Prediction of drug action: Elimination of error through emotionality, *Proc. 75th Ann. Conv. APA* **2**:69-70.

Powell, B. J., 1970, Alcohol effects on reversal learning in the Maudsley MR and MNR strains, *Proc. 78th Ann. Conv. APA* **5**:825-826.

Powell, B. J., and Hopper, D. J., 1971, Effects of strain differences and D-amphetamine sulfate on avoidance performance, *Psychonom. Sci.* **22**:167-170.

Powell, B. J., Martin, L. K., and Kamano, D. K., 1967, Relationship between emotionality, drug effects, and avoidance responses in Tryon S_1 and S_3 strains, *Can. J. Psychol.* **21**: 294-300.

Rambert, F. A., Amalvit, S., and Duteil, J., 1976, Problèmes posés par le choix d'une souche de souris pour l'etude des anxiolytiques, *J. Pharmacol.* **7**:517-530.

Randall, C. L., and Lester, D., 1974, Differential effects of ethanol and pentobarbital on sleep times in C57BL and BALB mice, *J. Pharm. Exp. Therap.* **188**:27-33.

Randall, C. L., and Lester, D., 1975*a*, Alcohol selection by DBA and C57BL mice arising from ova transfers, *Nature (London)* **255**:147-148.

Randall, C. L., and Lester, D., 1975*b*, Cross-fostering of DBA and C57B1 mice: Increase in voluntary consumption of alcohol by DBA weanlings, *J. Stud. Alcohol* **36**:973-980.

Randall, C. L., and Lester, D., 1975*c*, Social modification of alcohol consumption in inbred mice, *Science* **189**:149-151.

Randall, C. L., Carpenter, J. A., Lester, D., and Friedman, H. J., 1975, Ethanol-induced mouse strain differences in locomotor activity, *Pharmacol. Biochem. Behav.* **3**:533-535.

Randt, C. T., Barnett, B. M., McEwen, B. S., and Quartermain, D., 1971, Amnesic effects of cycloheximide on two strains of mice with different memory characteristics, *Exp. Neurol.* **30**:467-474.

Randt, C. T., Korein, J., and Levidow, L., 1973, Localization of action of two amnesia producing drugs in freely moving mice, *Exp. Neurol.* **41**:628-634.

Reed, T. E., 1976, Heritability of responses to alcohol in a heterogeneous mouse strain, *Behav. Genet.* **6**:114-115 (abstract).

Reinhard, J. F., Kosersky, D. S., and Peterson, G. R., 1976, Strain-dependent differences in responses to chronic administration of morphine: Lack of relationship to brain catecholamine levels in mice, *Life Sci.* **19**:1413-1420.

Remington, G., and Anisman, H., 1976, Genetic and ontogenetic variations in activity levels following treatment with scopolamine or D-amphetamine, *Develop. Psychobiol.* **9**:579-585.

Richardson, D., Karczmar, A. G., and Scudder, C. L., 1972, Intergeneric behavioral differences among methamphetamine treated mice, *Psychopharmacologia* **25**:347-375.

Riley, E. P., Freed, E. X., and Lester, D., 1976, Selective breeding of rats for differences in reactivity to alcohol; an approach to an animal model of alcoholism. I. General procedures, *J. Stud. Alcohol* **37**:1535-1547.

Riley, E. P., Worsham, E. D., Lester, D., and Freed, E. X., 1977, Selective breeding of rats for differences in reactivity to alcohol; an approach to an animal model of alcoholism. II. Behavioral measures, *J. Stud. Alcohol* **38:** 1705-1717.

Robustelli, F., 1966, Axione della nicotina sul condizionamento di salvaguardi di ratti di un mese (Action of nicotine on avoidance conditioning in month-old rats), *Rend. Accad. Lincei (Classe di Scienze fisiche, matematiche e naturali)* **40**:490-497.

Roderick, T. H., 1960, Selection for cholinesterase activity in the cerebral cortex of the rat, *Genetics* **45**:1123-1140.

Rodgers, D. A., 1966, Factors underlying differences in alcohol preference among inbred strains of mice, *Psychosom. Med.* **28**:498-513.

Rodgers, D. A., 1967, Alcohol preference in mice, in: *Comparative Psychopathology—Animal and Human* (J. Zubin and H. F. Hunt, eds.), pp. 184-201, Grune and Stratton, New York.

Rodgers, D. A., 1972a, Factors underlying differences in alcohol preference in inbred strains of mice, in: *The Biology of Alcoholism,* Vol. 2, *Physiology and Behavior* (B. Kissen and H. Begleiter, eds.), pp. 107-130, Plenum Press, New York.

Rodgers, D. A., 1972b, Inherited characteristics of inbred mice as these relate to voluntary alcohol consumption, in: *International Symposium on the Biological Aspects of Alcohol Consumption, 27-29 September 1971, Helsinki,* Vol. 20, pp. 105-112, The Finnish Foundation for Alcohol Studies, Helsinki.

Rodgers, D. A., and McClearn, G. E., 1962a, Alcohol preference of mice, in: *Roots of Behavior* (E. L. Bliss, ed.), pp. 68-95, Harper Bros., New York.

Rodgers, D. A., and McClearn, G. E., 1962b, Mouse strain differences in preference for various concentrations of alcohol, *Q. J. Stud. Alcohol.* **23**:26-33.

Rosecrans, J. A., and Schechter, M. D., 1972, Brain area nicotine levels in male and female rats of two strains, *Arch. Int. Pharmacodyn.* **196**:46-54.

Rosenzweig, M. R., 1964, Effects of heredity and environment on brain chemistry, brain anatomy, and learning ability in the rat, in: *Physiological Determinants of Behavior: Implications for Mental Retardation,* Vol. 14, pp. 3-40, University of Kansas Symposia.

Ross, R. B., 1964, Effects of strychnine sulphate on maze learning in rats, *Nature (London)* **201**:109-110.

Rush, W. A., and King, R. A., 1976, Effect of the albino gene upon sleep time in mice, *Behav. Genet.* **6**:116 (abstract).

Rusi, M., Eriksson, K., and Maki, J., 1977, Genetic differences in the susceptibility to acute ethanol intoxication in selected rat strains, in: *Alcohol Intoxication and Withdrawal Experimental Studies*, Vol. III (M. M. Gross, ed.), pp. 97-109, Plenum Press, New York.

Russell, D. E., and Stern, M. H., 1973, Sex and strain as factors in voluntary alcohol intake, *Physiol. Behav.* **10**:641-642.

Sanders, B., 1976, Sensitivity to low doses of ethanol and pentobarbital in mice selected for sensitivity to hypnotic doses of ethanol, *J. Comp. Physiol. Psychol.* **90**:394-398.

Sansone, M., and Messeri, P., 1974, Strain differences on the effects of chlordiazepoxide and chlorpromazine in avoidance behaviour of mice, *Pharmacol. Res. Commun.* **6**:179-185.

Santos, C. A., III, Middaugh, L., Buckholtz, N., and Zemp, J. W., 1973, Effects of methadone on activity and on brain monoamines in two mouse strains, *Fed. Proc., Fed. Am. Soc. Exp. Biol.* **32**:758 (abstract).

Satinder, K. P., 1971, Genotype-dependent effects of D-amphetamine sulfate and caffeine on escape–avoidance behavior in rats, *J. Comp. Physiol. Psychol.* **76**:359-364.

Satinder, K. P., 1972*a*, Behavior-genetic-dependent self-selection of alcohol in rats, *J. Comp. Physiol. Psychol.* **80**:422-434.

Satinder, K. P., 1972*b*, Effects of intertrial crossing punishment and *d*-amphetamine sulfate on avoidance and activity in four selectively bred rat strains, *Psychon. Sci.* **29**:291-293.

Satinder, K. P., 1975, Interactions of age, sex and long-term alcohol intake in selectively bred strains of rat, *J. Stud. Alcohol.* **36**:1493-1507.

Satinder, K. P., 1976, Differential effects of morphine on two -way avoidance in selectively bred rat strains, *Psychopharmacology,* **48**:235-237.

Satinder, K. P., 1977*a*, Oral intake of morphine in selectively bred rats, *Pharmacol. Biochem. Behav.* **7**:43-49.

Satinder, K. P., 1977*b*, Arousal explains difference in avoidance learning of genetically selected rat strains, *J. Comp. Physiol. Psychol.* **91**:1326-1336.

Satinder, K. P., and Petryshyn, W. R., 1974, Interaction between genotype, unconditioned stimulus, *d*-amphetamine and one-way avoidance behavior of rats, *J. Comp. Physiol. Psychol.* **86**:1059-1073.

Satinder, K. P., Royce, J. R., and Yeudall, L. T., 1970, Effects of electric shock, *d*-amphetamine sulphate, and chlorpromazine on factors of emotionality in inbred mice, *J. Comp. Physiol. Psychol.* **71**:443-447.

Schlesinger, K., 1966, Genetic and biochemical correlates of alcohol preference in mice, *Am. J. Psychiat.* **122**:767-773.

Schlesinger, K., and Griek, B. J., 1970, The genetics and biochemistry of audiogenic seizures, in: *Contributions to Behavior–Genetic Analysis: The Mouse as a Prototype* (G. Lindzey and D. D. Thiessen, eds.), pp. 219-257, Appleton-Century-Crofts, New York.

Schlesinger, K., and Sharpless, S. K., 1975, Audiogenic seizures and acoustic priming, in: *Psychopharmacogenetics* (B. E. Eleftheriou, ed.), pp. 383-433, Plenum Press, New York.

Schlesinger, K., Schreiber, R. A., and Pryor, G. T., 1968*a* Effects of *p*-chlorophenylalanine on conditioned avoidance learning, *Psychon. Sci.* **11**:225-226

Schlesinger, K., Boggan, W., and Freedman, D. X., 1968*b*, Genetics of audiogenic seizures. II. Effects of pharmacological manipulation of brain serotonin, norepinephrine and gamma-amino-butyric acid, *Life Sci.* **7**:437-447 (sic). (N.B. These page numbers repeated in this volume.)

Schlesinger, K., Boggan, W. O., and Griek, B. J., 1968*c*, Pharmacogenetic correlates of pentylenetetrazol and electronconvulsive seizure thresholds in mice, *Psychopharmacologia* **13**:181-188.

Schneider, C. W., Evans, S. K., Chenoweth, M. B., and Beman, F. L., 1973, Ethanol preference and behavioral tolerance in mice: Biochemical and neurophysiological mechanisms, *J. Comp. Physiol. Psychol.* **82**:466-474.

Schneider, C. W., Trzil, P., and D'Andrea, R., 1974, Neural tolerance in high and low ethanol selecting mouse strains, *Pharmacol. Biochem. Behav.* **2**:549-551.

Scott, J. P., 1974, Effects of psychotropic drugs on separation distress in dogs, in: *Neuropsychopharmacology, Proceedings of IX Congress of Collegium Internationale Neuropsychopharmacologicum, Paris, 7-12 July 1974, Int. Congr. Ser.* **359**: 735-745.

Scott, J. P., and Fuller, J. L., 1965, *Genetics and the Social Behavior of the Dog,* University of Chicago Press, Illinois.

Scott, J. P., Lee, C. T., and Ho, J. E., 1971, Effects of fighting, genotype and amphetamine sulfate on body temperature of mice, *J. Comp. Physiol. Psychol.* **76**:349-352.

Segovia–Riquelme, N., Campos, I., Solodkowska, W., Gonzales, G., Alvarado, R., and Mardones, J., 1962, Metabolism of labeled ethanol, acetate, pyruvate, and butyrate in "drinker" and "nondrinker" rats, *J. Biol. Chem.* **237**:2038-2040.

Segovia-Riquelme, N., Campos, I., Solodkowska, W., Figuerola-Camps, I., and Mardones, J., 1964, Glucose and gluconate metabolism in "drinker" and "nondrinker" rats, *Med. Exp.* **11**:185-190.

Segovia-Riquelme, N., Varela, A., and Mardones, J., 1971, Appetite for alcohol, in: *Biological Basis of Alcoholism* (Y. Israel and J. Mardones, eds.), pp. 299-334, Wiley, New York.

Seiden, L. S., and Peterson, D. D., 1968, Reversal of the reserpine-induced suppression of the conditioned-avoidance response by L-dopa: Correlation of behavioral and biochemical differences in two strains of mice, *J. Pharmacol. Exp. Ther.* **159**:422-428.

Sheppard, J. R., Albersheim, P., and McClearn, G., 1970, Aldehyde dehydrogenase and ethanol preference in mice, *J. Biol. Chem.* **245**:2876-2882.

Shuster, L., 1975, Genetic analysis of morphine effects: Activity, analgesia, tolerance and sensitization, in: *Psychopharmacogenetics* (B. E. Eleftheriou, ed.), pp. 73-97, Plenum Press, New York.

Shuster, L., Webster, G. W., and Yu, G., 1975a, Increased running response to morphine in morphine-pretreated mice, *J. Pharmacol. Exp. Ther.* **192**:64-72.

Shuster, L., Webster, G. W., Yu, G., and Eleftheriou, B. E., 1975b, A genetic analysis of the response to morphine in mice: Analgesia and running, *Psychopharmacologia* **42**:249-254.

Siemens, A. J., and Chan, A. W. K., 1975, Effects of pentobarbital in mice selectively bred for different sensitivities to ethanol, *Pharmacologist* **17**:197 (abstract).

Silverman, A. P., 1971, Behaviour of rats given a 'smoking dose' of nicotine, *Anim. Behav.* **19**: 67-74.

Simmel, E. C., 1976, Behavior genetic analysis of exploratory behavior and activity through use of recombinant inbred strains of mice: A progress report, *Behav. Genet.* **6**:117-118 (abstract).

Sinclair, J. D., 1974a, Lithium-induced suppression of alcohol drinking by rats, *Med. Biol.* **52**:133-136.

Sinclair, J. D., 1974b, Rats learning to work for alcohol, *Nature (London)* **249**:590-591.

Sinclair, J. D., Adkins, S., and Walker, D., 1973, Morphine-induced suppression of voluntary alcohol drinking in rats, *Nature (London)* **246**:425-426.

Singh, S. D., 1961, Conditioned emotional response in the rat: Effects of stimulant and depressant drugs, *J. Psychol. Res.* **5**(3):1-11.

Singh, S. D., and Eysenck, H. J., 1960, Conditioned emotional response in the rat. III. Drug antagonism, *J. Genet. Psychol.* **63**:275-285.

Sinha, S. N., Franks, C. M., and Broadhurst, P. L., 1958, The effect of a stimulant and a depressant drug on a measure of reactive inhibition, *J. Exp. Psychol.* **56**:349-354.

Soušková, M., and Benešová, O., 1963, The effect of chlorpromazine, phenmetrazine, imipramine and physostigmine on the exploratory reaction in rats with different excitability of the central nervous system, *Biochem. Pharmacol.* **12**:27 (abstract).

Sprott, R. L., and Staats, J., 1975, Behavioral studies using genetically defined mice: A bibliography, *Behav. Genet.* **5**:27-82.

Stasik, J. H., and Kidwell, J. F., 1969, Genotype, LSD and T-maze learning in mice, *Nature (London)* **224**:1224-1225.

Strange, A. W., Schneider, C. W., and Goldbort, R., 1976, Selection of C_3 alcohols by high and low selecting mouse strains and the effects on open field activity, *Pharmacol. Biochem. Behav.* **4**:527-530.

Stratton, L. O., and Petrinovich. L. F., 1963, Posttrial injections of an anticholinesterase drug on maze learning in two strains of rats, *Psychopharmacologia* **5**:47-54.

Taylor, B. A., 1976, Development of recombinant inbred lines of mice, *Behav. Genet.* **6**:118 (abstract).

Thiessen, D. D., 1964, Amphetamine toxicity, population density, and behavior: A review, *Psychol. Bull.* **62**:401-410.

Thiessen, D. D., Schlesinger, K., and Calhoun, W. H., 1961, Better learning: Neural enhancement or reduced interference? *Psychol. Rep.* **9**:493-496.

Thomas, K., 1969, Selection and avoidance of alcohol solutions by two strains of inbred mice and derived generations, *Q. J. Stud. Alcohol* **30**:849-861.

Thurman, R. G., and Pathman, D. E., 1975, Withdrawal symptoms from ethanol: Evidence against the involvement of acetaldehyde, in: *The Role of Acetaldehyde in the Actions of Ethanol,* Vol. 23 (K. O. Lindros and C. J. P. Eriksson, eds.), pp. 217-232, The Finnish Foundation for Alcohol Studies, Helsinki.

Tilson, H. A., and Rech, R. H., 1974, The effects of *p*-chlorophenylalanine on morphine analgesia, tolerance and dependence development in two strains of rats, *Psychopharmacologia* **35**:45-60.

Tilson, H. A., Maisel, A. S., Jourdan, M. G., and Rech, R. H., 1975, Comparison of the effects of *d*-amphetamine and lysergic acid diethylamide in two strains of rats having different behavioral baselines, *Behav. Biol.* **17**:463-471.

Tryon, R. C., 1931, Studies in individual differences in maze ability: IV. The constancy of individual differences: Correlation between learning and relearning, *J. Comp. Psychol.* **12**:303-345.

Tryon, R. C., 1940, Genetic differences in maze learning ability in rats, *Yearb. Nat. Soc. Stud. Educ.* **39**(1):111-119.

Tryon, R. C., 1942, Individual differences, in: *Comparative Psychology,* 2nd ed. (F. A. Moss, ed.), pp. 330-365, Prentice Hall, New York.

van Abeelen, J. H. F., 1966, Chlorpromazine and fur shaking in mice, *Experientia* **22**:360-361.

van Abeelen, J. H. F., 1970, Genetics of rearing behavior in mice, *Behav. Genet.* **1**:71-76.

van Abeelen, J. H. F., 1974, Genotype and the cholinergic control of exploratory behaviour in mice, in: *Genetics of Behaviour* (J. H. F. van Abeelen, ed.), pp. 347-374, North Holland Publishing Co., Amsterdam.

van Abeelen, J. H. F., and Strijbosch, H., 1969, Genotype-dependent effects of scopolamine and eserine on exploratory behaviour in mice, *Psychopharmacologia* **16**:81-88.

van Abeelen, J. H. F., Smits, A. J. M., and Raaijmakers, W. G. M., 1971, Central location of a genotype-dependent cholinergic mechanism controlling exploratory behaviour in mice, *Psychopharmacologia* **19**:324-328.

van Abeelen, J. H. F., Gilissen, L., Hanssen, T., and Lenders, A., 1972, Effects of intra-hippocampal injections with methylscopolamine and neostigmine upon exploratory behaviour in two inbred mouse strains, *Psychopharmacologia* **24**:470-475.

van Abeelen, J. H. F., Daems, J., and Douma, G., 1973, Memory storage in three inbred mouse strains after injection of cycloheximide, *Physiol. Behav.* **10**:751-753.

van Abeelen, J. H. F., Ellenbroek, G. A., and Wigman, H. G. A. J., 1975, Exploratory behaviour in two selectively-bred lines of mice after intraphippocampal injection of methylscopolamine, *Psychopharmacologia* **41**:111-112.

Vander Vliet, G., and Crumpacker, D. W., 1976, Drug-induced sleep time in F_1 hybrids of short-sleep and long-sleep mouse lines, *Behav. Genet.* **6**:119 (abstract).

Vesell, E. S., 1968, Genetic and environmental factors affecting hexobarbital metabolism in mice, *Ann. N. Y. Acad. Sci.* **151**:900-902.

Vesell, E. S., 1975, Pharmacogenetics, *Biochem. Pharmacol.* **24**:445-450.

Vesell, E. S., Lang, C. M., White, W. J., Passananti, G. T., Hill, R. N., Clemens, T. L., Liu, D. K., and Johnson, W. D., 1976, Environmental and genetic factors affecting the response of laboratory animals to drugs, *Fed. Proc., Fed. Am. Soc. Exp. Biol.* **35**:1125-1132.

Votava, Z., and Soušková, M., 1965, Research on the psychotropic drugs using the exploratory reaction method in rats with different levels of excitability, in: *Pharmacology of Conditioning, Learning and Retention* (M. Ya. Mikhelson and V. G. Longo, eds.), pp. 67-73, Pergamon, Oxford. (*Proceedings of the 2nd International Pharmacological Meeting*, Prague 1963, Vol. 1.)

Wallgren, H., 1959, Sex difference in ethanol tolerance of rats, *Nature (London)* **184**:726-727.

Wallgren, H., and Barry, H. III., 1970, *Actions of Alcohol,* Vol. 1, *Biochemical Physiological and Psychological Aspects.* Vol. II, *Chronic and Clinical Aspects,* Elsevier, Amsterdam.

Watson, R. H. J., 1960, Constitutional differences between two strains of rats with different behavioural characteristics, in: *Symposium of 4th European Conference on Psychosomatic Research, Hamburg, April 1959* (A. Jores and H. Freyberger, eds.), pp. 160-165, Karger, Basel.

Way, E.L., Loh, H.H., and Shea, F.H., 1969, Simultaneous quantitative assessment of morphine tolerance and physical dependence, *J. Pharmacol. Exp. Ther.* **167**:1-8.

Werboff, J., Anderson, A., and Ross, S., 1967, Mice of a four-way cross: Coat color associated with behavior and response to *d*-amphetamine, *J. Psychol.* **66**:99-117.

Westbrook, W. H., and McGaugh, J. L., 1964, Drug facilitation of latent learning, *Psychopharmacologia* **5**:440-446.

Whitman, J. R., and Peretz, E., 1969, The effects of nembutal on the estrous activity cycle, *Physiol. Behav.* **4**:963-964.

Whitney, G., 1972, Relationship between alcohol preference and other behaviors in laboratory mice, in: *International Symposium on the Biological Aspects of Alcohol Consumption, 27-29 September 1971, Helsinki,* Vol. 20. (O. A. Forsander and K. Eriksson, eds.), pp. 151-161, The Finnish Foundation for Alcohol Studies, Helsinki.

Whitney, G., McClearn, G. E., and DeFries, J. C., 1970, Heritability of alcohol preference in laboratory mice and rats, *J. Hered.* **61**:165-169.

Whitney, G., Horowitz, G. P., and Collins, R. L., 1977, Relationship between morphine self-administration and the effect of morphine across strains of mice, *Behav. Genet.* **7**:92 (abstract).

Wilcock, J., 1969, Gene action and behavior: an evaluation of major gene pleiotropism, *Psychol. Bull.* **72**:1-29.

Wilcock, J., and Fulker, D. W., 1973, Avoidance learning in rats: Genetic evidence for two distinct behavioral processes in the shuttle-box, *J. Comp. Physiol. Psychol.* **82**:247-253.

Wimer, R. E., 1968, Bases of a facilitative effect upon retention resulting from posttrial etherization, *J. Comp. Physiol. Psychol.* **65**:340-342.

Wimer, R. E., 1973, Dissociation of a phenotypic correlation: Response to post-trial etherization and to variation in temporal distribution of practice trials, *Behav. Genet.* **3**:379-386.

Wimer, R. E., Symington, L., Farmer, H., and Schwartzkroin, P., 1968, Differences in memory processes between inbred mouse strains C57BL/6J and DBA/2J, *J. Comp. Physiol. Psychol.* **65**:126-131.

Wise, R. A., 1974, Strain and supplier differences affecting ethanol intake by rats, *Q. J. Stud. Alcohol* **35**:667-669.

Worsham, F. D., Riley, E. P., Anandam, N., Lister, P., Freed, E. X., and Lester, D., 1977, Selective breeding of rats for differences in reactivity to alcohol: An approach to an animal model of alcoholism. III. Some physical and behavioral measures, in: *Alcohol Intoxication and Withdrawal,* Vol. IIIa (M. M. Gross, ed.), pp. 71-81, Plenum Press, New York.

Wraight, K. B., Weldon, E., Gupta, B. D., and Holland, H. C., 1967, The effects of post-trial injections of nicotine on the learning of an underwater discrimination task by rats, *Anim. Behav.* **15**:287-290.

Wright, D. C., 1974, Differentiating stimulus and storage hypotheses of state-dependent learning, *Fed. Proc., Fed. Am. Soc. Exp. Biol.* **33**:1797-1799.

Yanai, J., and Ginsburg, B. E., 1973, The effect of alcohol consumed by parent mice on the susceptibility to audiogenic seizure and the open-field behavior of their offspring, *Behav. Genet.* **3**:418 (abstract).

Yanai, J., and Ginsburg, B. E., 1976, Increased sensitivity to chronic ethanol in isolated mice, *Psychopharmacologia* **46**:185-189.

Yanai, J., Sze, P. Y., and Ginsburg, B. E., 1975, Differential induction of behavioral and metabolic changes by ethanol during early development, *Behav. Genet.* **5**:111-112 (abstract).

Yanai, J., Ginsburg, B. E., and Vinopal, B., 1976, Comparison of early effects of ethanol on agonistic behavior in inbred strains of mice, *Behav. Genet.* **6**:122-123 (abstract).

Author Index

Boldface page numbers indicate the location of a reference including the name.

Subject Index